Who Survives Cancer?

Who Survives Cancer?

Howard P. Greenwald

UNIVERSITY OF CALIFORNIA PRESS

Berkeley / Los Angeles / Oxford

University of California Press
Berkeley and Los Angeles, California

University of California Press, Ltd.
Oxford, England

Library of Congress Cataloging-in-Publication Data

Greenwald, Howard P.
  Who survives cancer? / Howard P. Greenwald.
    p.   cm.
  Includes bibliographical references and index.
  ISBN 0-520-07725-3 (cloth : alk. paper). — ISBN 0-520-07729-6
(pbk.: alk. paper)
    1. Cancer—Prognosis.   2. Cancer—Social aspects.   3. Cancer—
Psychological aspects.   4. Cancer—Patients.   I. Title.
    [DNLM: 1. Health Maintenance Organizations—United States.
2. Health Services—organization & administration—United States.
3. Neoplasms—mortality—United States.   4. Neoplasms—
prevention & control—United States.   5. Neoplasms—therapy.
6. Survival Rate—United States.   QZ 200 G816w]
  RC262.G736   1992
  362.1'96994—dc20
  DNLM/DLC
  for Library of Congress   91-36909

Printed in the United States of America

9 8 7 6 5 4 3 2 1

The paper used in this publication meets the minimum requirements
of American National Standard for Information Sciences—
Permanence of Paper for Printed Library Materials, ANSI
Z39.48-1984 ⊗

To my parents

Contents

List of Figures

List of Tables

Preface

*When they arrived in Athens, though a few had houses of their
own to go to, or could find an asylum with friends or relatives, by
far the greater number had to take up their dwelling in the parts
of the city that were not built over and in the temples and chapels of
the heroes. . . . The occupation of the plot of ground lying below the
citadel called the Pelasgian had been forbidden by a curse; and
there was an ominous fragment of a Pythian oracle which said*

Leave the Pelasgian parcel desolate,
Woe worth the day that men inhabit it!

*Yet this too was now built over in the necessity of the moment. And
in my opinion, if the oracle proved true, it was in the opposite sense
to what was expected. For the misfortunes of the state did not arise
from the unlawful occupation, but the necessity of the occupation
from the war; and though the god did not mention this, he foresaw
that it would be an evil day for Athens in which the plot came to be
inhabited.*

—Thucydides

The ancient Greek historian Thucydides knew that social
and economic conditions can determine the health and illness of a
people. This quotation from *The Peloponnesian War* reflects a profound
awareness that the state of society may become a life-or-death matter. In
the darkest days of that war, Sparta laid siege to Athens. Athenians from
the countryside, forced to take refuge within the city's walls, soon began

to sicken and die. A monstrous epidemic enveloped the city. Contemporary Athenians attributed the calamity to violation of sacred places by the newcomers. But Thucydides, the first "social epidemiologist," thought otherwise. His chronicle suggests that war, siege, and the crowding together of people in all available space gave rise to the uncontrollable plague.

Many view cancer as the plague of modern times. Like epidemics of past ages, cancer defies the efforts of the best physicians to cure the patient or prolong his or her life. As their forebears viewed other disease, people in the modern world view cancer with a special degree of terror. And people today explain this disease in spiritual terms, seeking the cause of illness in the individual's personal outlook, spirit, or life force. In this respect, today's spiritualists are no less in error than the ancient Greeks.

This book shares the widely held view of cancer as a fearsome disease that often resists our best technical capabilities. But in its analysis of survival, it adopts a position akin to that of the ancient Greek historian, seeking much of the explanation in concrete, worldly terms. It concentrates on resources and conditions that affect the individual's ability to have his or her illness detected and to obtain appropriate care in a timely manner. All things being equal, these factors make the real difference in survival.

Important personal resources may include tangible ones such as income and wealth, or intangibles such as education and culture. Conditions completely outside the individual are crucial, particularly the existence of technically capable, efficiently organized, and accessible health care professionals. Examination of these and related social resources has become increasingly important as public generosity declined in the late twentieth century. These years saw the welfare state increasingly come into question. Government and industry became more hesitant about covering the citizen's or worker's health care needs. Individuals themselves turned their attention from caring for others and planning for the future to personal rewards and immediate consumption. Examination of recent developments in public and private health care and their possible effects on the survival chances of individual cancer patients helps identify concerns that must be shared by society as a whole. As was true in the war among the ancient Greeks, a crisis in the nation's health raises issues of even more general significance.

The present volume owes its existence to a series of accidents and the availability of resources initially allocated for other purposes. During the early 1980s, I enjoyed the privilege of managing a large-scale project for Dr. John J. Bonica, chairman emeritus of the Department of Anesthesiology at the University of Washington. A pioneer in the study of pain associated with cancer, Bonica had alerted the National Cancer Institute to the importance of performing a study of pain among cancer patients based on a survey of individuals in a defined geographical area. Previous studies had been largely confined to single hospitals or treatment centers, and thus could not be assumed to represent the broad range of persons recently treated for cancer in the community.

In addition to funds, Dr. Bonica's leadership helped secure two crucial resources: access to the Cancer Surveillance System (CSS), a population-based tumor registry at the Fred Hutchinson Cancer Research Center in Seattle, and to cancer patients themselves. The pain study identified and interviewed patients throughout the Seattle metropolitan area. As a junior investigator, I doubt that I could have obtained the funding, use of the CSS, or access to patients on my own in the highly competitive world of cancer research. Completed in 1983, the pain study is now part of the clinical literature on cancer.[1]

In order to assess fully the pain problems of individuals, the study collected a broad range of data on each. In addition to clinical data, basic demographics, and some information on source of care from the CSS, we obtained histories of each patient's awareness of becoming ill and level of personal resources. Also, using standardized questions and tests, we assessed each individual's emotional state, physical function, and, of course, pain. In visits lasting up to four hours, interviewers personally questioned a large number of cancer patients, inquiring in detail about their illness and its treatment. To update information on the patients' condition and care, investigators often visited them repeatedly. The resulting array of facts provided an unusually detailed picture of the patient's illness and his or her pattern of responses to it. It was clear that such information could help us answer many questions about cancer patients in addition to assessing their pain problems.

I first focused on the ability of employed individuals to continue working after they contracted cancer. A grant from the American Cancer Society enabled me to pursue this research, the findings from which have been published elsewhere.[2] This grant gave me the opportunity to become more familiar with the data and to augment them with information on occupations from other studies.

From the very beginning, I had suspected that the cancer patient's experience might be useful in assessing changes in the health care system that were commencing just at the time of the study's inception. Detection and survival of serious disease, after all, are among the most important "products" the consumer seeks in health care. A significant percentage of the patients surveyed paid for at least some of their care from personal income and savings. While insurance from employers or government agencies had been increasingly generous throughout the mid-century, the trend was just beginning to reverse. A major prepaid group practice, or health maintenance organization (HMO), already operated in the Seattle area, and many of the surveyed patients obtained their care from it. While HMOs were rare in most parts of the United States before the 1980s, they proliferated rapidly as the decade wore on.

As projects were begun and completed, it became apparent that the detailed information on patients in the pain study could shed an unusually bright light on the determinants of survival. Through the CSS, which continuously monitors surviving cancer patients, I regularly added information on patient survival through mid-1987, updating records on all survivors for at least five years. In the original face-to-face interviews, individuals were asked where they received their health care and whether out-of-pocket payments had been required. Public information sources such as the U.S. Census provided additional data. I have called the product of this accumulation of facts the Seattle Longitudinal Assessment of Cancer Survival, or SLACS. Other scientists have studied the relationships of organization and finance to health care outcomes, but usually they have not concentrated on populations with serious, immediate needs and have not considered many of the important background factors represented here. Others have examined the effects of personal resources and social status on cancer survival, but lacked the direct, in-depth contact with cancer patients afforded by the SLACS.

This book addresses several distinct aspects of health care and the quality of life in the United States. As suggested above, it provides information about the impacts of changes in the health care system that occurred in the 1980s. Cancer detection and survival are potentially important indicators of these impacts. Closely related to this purpose is the reporting of relations between these indicators of the quality of care and personal resources. Studies have appeared on changes in access to care by distinct groups, such as the elderly and the poor, but not on the outcomes of care for those suffering from a specific condition requiring the immediate application of appropriate interventions. These are the conditions under which the health care system and the accompanying "social safety net" meet their most meaningful tests.

Of equal importance, this book provides information useful to those specifically concerned with cancer survival. Two important issues receive special attention. Most citizens of the modern world look to progress in cancer research in hopes of a cure for the dread disease. Reviewing this progress over the past thirty years, this book develops a realistic perspective on prospects for cure. A number of prominent writers assert that mood and outlook on life affect cancer survival. Using the rich data base from the SLACS, this book includes an examination of psychological variables as survival prognosticators. Although such variables have been the subject of much writing and some scientific studies, perhaps no previous investigation has assessed factors such as mood state and emotional dysfunction as systematically, and monitored survival as long, as the one reported here.

I hope that many individuals will benefit from this book. The information in it can make health care professionals—including physicians, nurses, clinical psychologists, social workers, and administrators— aware of factors often untouched in biomedical and administrative training that may prove crucial to the survival of cancer patients. For people in positions that influence the lives of health professionals and patients alike—that is, the policymakers of health care—this book provides clues to outcomes of some of the most important policy decisions being made today by corporations and government agencies. This study also will aid individuals concerned with reducing the threat that cancer poses to their personal survival. Though not a prescription for action, it may serve as a means of analyzing one's health care resources and the risks associated with their level and configuration. Finally, this book will prove highly useful to students in all areas wishing to learn more about the United States health care system: its structure, recent changes, and performance.

Each reader will encounter special challenges. The material presented cuts across several disciplines and hence conforms perfectly to the methodological teachings of none. Accustomed to the traditional experimental method, physicians and biomedical scientists may object to the use of multivariate statistics to model survival. Psychologists may demand more direct assessment of emotional states, economists more complete enumeration of individual resources. The general reader may hesitate to take up a book that is not devoted mainly to anecdotes about personal experience and tales about triumphs over cancer. Specialists in all disciplines are likely to encounter some material that appears elementary and some that is unfamiliar.

But everyone should exercise the patience and flexibility required to answer the important questions posed here. Objective, systematic analysis cannot depend entirely on anecdotes or case histories—the content of most popular books on cancer survival. Unlike new treatments or medications, hypotheses about the behavior of patients and the operation of health care systems cannot be tested in laboratories or through clinical experiments. The study reported here does not match the rigor of biomedical science, but is nevertheless systematic and objective. Meaningful answers to the questions posed require an interdisciplinary perspective. The pages that follow concentrate on reporting facts and figures, but do so in language and with illustrations comfortably accessible to the lay reader.

Chapter 1 provides a statement of the issues and an overview of recent changes in the health care system. Chapter 2 reviews the nature of cancer as a disease, suggests ways of assessing survival and cure, and considers whether cure is really an appropriate goal in cancer treatment. Chapter 3 provides basic information on cancer treatment, assesses the promise of cure in the near future, and evaluates the benefits of experimental and nonstandard interventions for individual patients. Focusing on prevention, Chapter 4 asks how much can be gained by taking steps to avoid contracting cancer. In Chapters 5 through 8, the SLACS findings are presented. Chapter 5 provides a systematic analysis of whether favorable mood states and normal emotional functioning promote cancer survival. Chapter 6 assesses the actual benefits of early cancer detection in promoting survival. Chapter 7 analyzes relationships between personal resources (such as income, wealth, and education) and health care outcomes (such as detection, treatment, and life expectancy). Chapter 8 focuses on the health maintenance organization (HMO), asking whether the striking change in medical service delivery it represents is likely to prove beneficial or detrimental to cancer patients of the future. Finally, Chapter 9 suggests strategies for the reduction of personal risks, draws policy implications for health care, and discusses issues that cancer raises about America's future as a community. Two technical appendices give additional detail on the SLACS and information on the statistical techniques and findings used in the study.

I would like to acknowledge the contributions several key institutions in the field of cancer research have made to my work. The National Cancer Institute funded the initial data collection effort as a study of cancer pain (Grant no. 5 R18 CA 32564-02). The American Cancer Society provided support for a study of work disability among cancer patients (Grant no. PBR-11), which enabled me to continue and extend the investigation to include additional treatment and quality-of-life issues. Further funding from the American Cancer Society (Grant no. PDT-393) will allow the study reported here to continue, generating more detailed information and more specific recommendations. The Fred Hutchinson Cancer Research Center in Seattle deserves special thanks for granting access to data from the CSS, without which the research leading to this book would have been impossible.

I acknowledge major debts to numerous colleagues who have assisted me in all phases of this work. John J. Bonica, M.D., deserves special thanks for his encouragement and for allowing me free access to data from the pain study. I am grateful to Susan J. Dirks, M.D., David Thomas, M.D., Berta Nicol, Chris Schwarz, and Mary Potts for their guidance and assistance in data collection and management. Drs. Ruth McCorkle, Curtis Henke, Edgar F. Borgatta, Lincoln Polissar, and Barbara Uenaka provided invaluable clinical information and methodological guidance. Drs. Steven A. Hart, Richard Ikeda, and Arnold Kaluzny provided material suggestions for improvement of the original manuscript. Drs. Edward Perrin, Anita Francis, and Marilyn Bergner made important contributions in the early phases of the foregoing research. Adina Katz, Kristine Mickus, Jeffrey Persson, Christina Paylunian, Leigha Krueger, and Deborah Dickstein deserve special thanks for assistance in research and manuscript preparation. The conclusions presented here are entirely mine.

Howard P. Greenwald
Seattle, 1991

CHAPTER ONE

The Problem and Its Context

Victory over cancer is not at hand. Of Americans who died in the mid-1980s, a greater proportion succumbed to cancer than in the 1930s. Individuals may take steps to reduce risk of the disease, but even the most knowledgeable and conscientious cannot protect themselves completely. Millions of Americans each year receive treatment for cancer. For the foreseeable future, a single factor—the timeliness and effectiveness of medical care—will determine their survival chances. The availability of such care reflects not only scientific knowledge and medical resources but also the general well-being of Americans as individuals and the quality of life in American society.

Since the 1930s, cancer research has enjoyed public support greater than any competing scientific enterprise except the development of military hardware. But dramatic increases in survival have come in only a few forms of cancer. In advanced malignancies, patients have only a slightly better chance of cure than they had a generation ago. Early detection may well have contributed more to survival than improvement in treatment has.

Few would argue that cancer research should not remain a major priority for public funding and private charity. Millions of Americans today qualify as "cancer survivors," having been cured of the disease or living with it in an arrested state. For many of these persons, even slight improvements in treatment have meant additional years of life. But for the average person with cancer, factors much less glamorous than science and research affect survival chances more directly. During the mid-

1

twentieth century, the growing availability of physician and hospital services to all patients doubtlessly increased cancer survival. As late as the 1930s, most Americans relied entirely on personal resources or private charity to pay medical and hospital bills. In the decades following World War II, "third-party payers"—private health insurance plans, nonprofit groups such as Blue Cross and Blue Shield, and traditional insurance carriers such as Aetna and Prudential—began covering the costs of more and more individuals seeking medical care. For employed individuals, medical benefits became broader with each succeeding year. In 1965, Congress enacted Medicare and Medicaid to support health care for the elderly and poor, programs that were expending close to $100 billion per year by the beginning of the 1980s. These developments substantially increased access to treatment for all medical conditions.

The impact of expanded access to health care was most visible among the disadvantaged. Large-scale, national studies monitored the utilization of health services by poor people and minority group members during the years following the inception of Medicare and Medicaid. Visits to physicians' offices and stays in hospitals rapidly increased among members of these traditionally disadvantaged groups. Of particular relevance to cancer survival, black women reported receiving the Pap test—a highly acclaimed early-detection procedure for cervical cancer—more often than white women in 1979. This finding reflected the closing of a major gap: black women had received the Pap test less frequently than white women as late as 1973.[1]

While expansion of access to health care may have reduced differences in survival chances, it did not erase them, as is illustrated by survival differences between blacks and whites for cervical cancer. A comparison of women diagnosed in the early 1960s with those diagnosed in the mid-1970s is most relevant. Medicare, Medicaid, and most private insurance plans grew swiftly in this era. In the early 1960s, the five-year survival rates were 58 percent for white women and 47 percent for black women; by the mid-1970s, the rates were 68 percent for white women and 64 percent for black women.[2] Five-year survival increased for both groups, and the gap between whites and blacks narrowed from eleven to four percentage points. Blacks, however, continued to have lower survival rates than whites. Other frequently diagnosed forms of cancer duplicate this picture.

These comparisons should alert all Americans to the importance of maintaining ready access to basic health care. But to most, the word *cancer* does not engender thoughts about everyday things like government programs or insurance. Blue Cross or Medicare becomes important to people when they or a member of their family contracts a serious illness. In most minds, the word *cancer* first conjures up the reasonable fear associated with a widespread, life-threatening illness. Further reflection tends to draw on our faith in technology and belief in the individual. The public most often looks to "scientific breakthroughs" to reduce the cancer threat; it attributes cancer's prevalence to alleged government and industrial insensitivity to environmental hazards; it identifies personal discouragement—"giving up on life"—as conducive to developing cancer and personal courage and positive thinking as important to survival. The predominance of these concerns in the public's thinking about cancer, however, appears inappropriate.

Our civilization believes in and expects continual technological breakthroughs. In fact, historians of science tell us that slow, methodical refinement of established knowledge and practice has as much impact on our lives as revolutionary theories and inventions. The fact that increases in cancer survival rates over the past fifty years have been slow and modest is consistent with this formulation. Typically, scientific discoveries reported in the mass media as breakthroughs turn out to be, at best, small steps forward.

Recent experience with experimental anticancer drugs illustrates the slowness and uncertainty of progress in cancer treatment. News reports in 1985 suggested that a drug called interleukin-2 (IL-2) could soon tip the balance in favor of even patients with previously incurable cancers. A year later, David Golde, chief of hematology and oncology at UCLA, called the publicity "so far out of proportion to the scientific development that it was almost incomprehensible." More recent tests of IL-2 have been promising, but they suggest a future use as an adjunct to conventional therapy rather than a revolutionary development in itself. A medication of somewhat earlier vintage, interferon, was originally billed as a cancer panacea; it is now used to treat only one very rare form of the disease.[3]

The presence of cancer-causing substances in foods, cosmetics, building materials, and industrial waste has focused public attention on the industries that manufacture these items and the government agencies responsible for monitoring them. Control of toxic waste ranks among the most important issues identified by respondents in recent public opinion polls. The public is reluctant to accept the introduction of *any* synthetic cancer-causing agent into the food supply or environment. Public law reflects this reluctance, banning the use of known carcinogens of any potency in foods and cosmetics.

But meticulous testing of a vast array of suspected man-made carcinogens reveals that most are no more hazardous than many natural substances. Beyond protection from a few obvious hazards—airborne asbestos, for instance—it appears unlikely that control of industrially produced chemicals can substantially reduce the average person's risk of cancer. The Environmental Protection Agency, for example, recently banned the use of EDB, a grain fumigant known to cause cancer. But naturally occurring chemicals in a single raw mushroom are 200 times more carcinogenic than the consumer's average daily intake of EDB from treated grain and grain products.[4]

Still, our culture places major responsibility on the individual. Most Americans would doubtless agree that individuals must share the blame for exposure to one of the most hazardous of the known carcinogens: tobacco tar. Until recently, self-exposure to this major cancer-causing substance was widely tolerated. In the past few years, public policy has begun to discourage smoking, by banning it from most parts of public buildings and conveyances. More important, social pressure against smoking has increased substantially. Prominent public health expert Lester Breslow recently remarked that ashtrays will be as rarely seen in a generation or so as spittoons are today. Holding individuals responsible for their health, a growing "health promotion and wellness" movement tends to view lack of knowledge and poor self-care as the principal causes of disease.

Consistent with this movement is an increasingly popular belief that the cancer patient's mood, emotional response, and fundamental personality traits play major roles in determining his or her survival.[5] This belief receives support from professionals in the emerging discipline of behavioral medicine. Psychologists and physicians in this field have identified ego strength,[6] will to live,[7] and other indicators of emotional well-being as harbingers of survival. Practitioners in this field have developed supportive therapy programs aimed at enhancing quality of life and increasing survival chances. O. C. Simonton, the best known of these practitioners, reports that patients who participated in a therapy program designed to reduce anxiety, hostility, and depression lived longer than those who did not participate.[8] Drawing on personal experience, Norman Cousins has popularized the notion that mood elevation through humor can cure dreaded disease.[9]

The value of interventions capable of improving the cancer patient's outlook on life needs no substantiation. The assertion that enhancement of emotional well-being can prolong the cancer patient's life, however, requires objective support based on valid measurement of emotional distress and experimentally sound comparisons of survival time of individuals with varying degrees of emotional disturbance. Few if any studies of this kind have been reported. Despite the popularity of their conviction, those who hold that emotional well-being or related interventions can promote survival among cancer patients have provided no proof.

The expectation of scientific breakthroughs, suspicion of man-made chemicals, and the belief that individuals are responsible for their own health are important elements in our culture of technology and individualism. Each of these elements has some basis in fact; related actions and public policies can undoubtedly reduce the risk of cancer and other dread disease. But the most favorable outcomes of clinical investigations currently in progress, the tightest control over the manufacture of chemical carcinogens, and the most conscientious individual behavior will not displace cancer as a major threat to life and well-being in modern society. People in all walks of life will continue to contract and die from cancer.

In the expectation that "science"—either medicine or toxicology—will not fundamentally alter this picture in the foreseeable future, this book evaluates the effects of nonbiomedical factors on the survival chances of cancer patients. Some of these factors are under the control of individuals themselves. Others are social in nature, promoting or inhibiting the ability of all individuals at risk of or actually diagnosed with cancer to take the most favorable actions. In most cases, these actions will focus on promoting timely access to competently applied, standard diagnostic and therapeutic services available in the community. Knowledge of these factors may guide individual actions—both the patient's and the professional's—to increase survival chances.

Second, this book raises issues about the "health care system," a complex network of health professionals, hospitals, laboratories, and corporations supported by insurance plans, government programs, and patient remittances. It asks whether recent changes in this system have begun to affect cancer survival. This question has significance far beyond cancer survival itself. Similar issues may be raised about heart disease, strokes, diabetes, and a number of other diseases which, though often treatable, kill many Americans every year. These questions bear on current dilemmas about the organization and delivery of health care in America.

Finally, this book examines differences in cancer survival as an issue intimately connected with the general quality of life in the United States today. It considers the relative importance of individual initiative versus social equity. It identifies trade-offs we may have to make between consuming on a personal level and contributing to collective resources in order to live long and truly well in the century to come. The question "Who survives cancer?" raises a fundamental question about the proper role for one of modern society's key institutions: the welfare state.

A Disease of Our Times

Cancer deserves special attention for several reasons. It is typical of "modern diseases," those that constitute the most important health problems in the late twentieth century.[10] These diseases tend to be chronic. Even if they end in death, they are not immediately life-threatening. They may develop over periods of years before producing visible signs or symptoms. Single, external agents (such as a bacterium or virus) are seldom identifiable as causes of these conditions. In these diseases, treatment often takes the form of repeated interventions using multiple approaches at various stages. Treatment often aims not at cure but at "management," by which health professionals attempt to achieve added months or years of survival with acceptable levels of comfort, alertness, and function. Speed of detection tends to be crucial, as does patient cooperation in detection and treatment. Steps taken by the patient may increase the likelihood of detection at a treatable stage. Long-term, self-motivated compliance with medical regimens may be necessary for treatment to be effective. Social and emotional factors are widely believed to influence development, detection, and cure.

The patterns of illness and responses effective against it have changed markedly over the past century. In the 1800s, epidemics of contagious disease still claimed many lives in Europe and America. Public health measures in the areas of quarantine and sanitation significantly reduced this hazard. At the beginning of the twentieth century, epidemics of contagious disease still occurred, but illnesses striking isolated individuals had become a more important cause of death.[11] Individual medical treatment began to supplant public health as the most frequent countermeasure. Such treatment utilized methods that appear straightforward by today's standards—chemical or antibiotic agents to prevent or cure bacterial or viral infections. Diseases of this kind were typically acute, patients either recovering or succumbing in short order. As of 1900, the three most frequent causes of death in the United States were pneumonia and influenza, tuberculosis, and acute intestinal disease (such as typhoid and diarrhea). In that year, 1,719 individuals out of every 100,000 died, these three conditions accounting for just under one-third of the deaths.[12]

By the late twentieth century, heart disease, cancer, and stroke had become the three leading causes of death in the United States. Reflecting a substantial increase in life expectancy since the turn of the century, the death rate itself had dropped to approximately 883 per 100,000, roughly half the figure recorded in 1900.[13] Public health measures and medical technology had all but eliminated the contagious, acute illnesses that had accounted for most mortality. The predominant remaining causes of mortality were "modern diseases." Heart disease, cancer, and stroke accounted for about two-thirds of all deaths by the 1980s. Most of the other causes of death were also modern diseases, including diabetes mellitus, cirrhosis of the liver, and arteriosclerosis.

The personal experiences of patients with these diseases have many similarities. Heart attack survivors, for example, typically receive treatment designed to minimize mortality hazard related to heart muscle damage and prevent or delay new heart attacks. The patient may receive both surgical and medical treatment, including bypass surgery to restore adequate circulation to the heart muscle and drugs to control blood pressure. Initial treatment of cancer is likely to include surgical intervention to remove detectable growths, followed by radiation or chemotherapy to destroy remaining malignant cells. Individuals with either disease are likely to need continuing care, at least some of it in the hospital, as new heart attacks occur or malignant tumors are found. The typical sequence of initial illness, treatment, recurrence, and retreatment stands in marked contrast to the acute diseases of the early twentieth century, in which survival of the initial illness episode usually meant freedom from further infection—unless the individual experienced renewed exposure from the outside.

But cancer differs from most other modern diseases in ways that make differences in survival chances especially revealing with respect to health and society. Deaths from most of the other such diseases are decreasing in number—especially deaths from heart disease.[14] Improved medical management of heart disease has played a part in controlling this major threat to survival, as a wide variety of drugs to control angina and metabolic precursors of acute attacks have become available. But of equal importance, individuals of all ages in the past generation have modified their lifestyles in a manner much less conducive to heart disease. Red meat and other high-cholesterol food products now occupy a smaller place in the American diet than they did only a few years ago. Regular physical exercise has become popular among a much broader segment of the population than in earlier generations. The belief that exercise is essential to health for persons of all ages has gained very wide acceptance.

Deaths from cancer, on the contrary, are increasing. The death rate from cancer among males in the early 1950s was about 170 per 100,000 individuals in the population; in the early 1980s, the rate was 216 per 100,000, representing an increase of 27 percent. The death rate *dropped* for females, from about 147 to 135 per 100,000, but by too small a percentage (about 8 percent) to offset the increase in the male death rate. For the population as a whole, the death rate from cancer rose from about 158 to 170 per 100,000. These comparisons take account of changes in the age distribution within the United States population over the decades.[15] The fact that Americans, on the average, are getting older does not explain the increased cancer death rate.[16]

A combination of rates of occurrence and chances for survival accounts for the death rate from any disease. As a disease becomes more frequent (i.e., as its *incidence* increases), the rate of death will increase unless its victims begin to survive longer or are more often cured. The death rate for lung cancer has increased because of a marked increase in incidence in the late twentieth century and a stubbornly low rate of recovery among its victims.

A large part of the increase in the cancer death rate unquestionably stems from a behavioral factor, increased cigarette smoking. As the rate of cigarette smoking increased in the population, deaths from lung cancer also increased. Cigarette smoking has increased most rapidly among females, who have also experienced the sharpest increase in deaths from lung cancer.

Little change has taken place in the death rates for most cancers in the past thirty years. After lung cancer, malignancies of the breast, colon and rectum, and prostate gland account for the lion's share of cancer deaths in the United States each year. A slight increase has occurred in the prostate cancer death rate. The rate for breast cancer has remained constant. While the death rate from colon and rectal cancer has declined for females, it has remained constant for males.[17]

The death rates for a few specific forms of the disease have declined. Acute leukemia has been a success story as a result of chemotherapy advances. Among the "solid tumors," mortality from cervical cancer decreased between 1950 and 1982. Improved treatment methods, including improved surgical procedures, account for part of this improvement. Early detection through the use of the Pap test, however, appears to have played a more important role. The proportion of cervical cancer patients surviving five years or longer increased markedly during the period.[18]

As in heart disease, individual behavior has unquestionably played a role in decreasing some cancer death rates. Strong evidence for a behavioral risk of contracting the disease, however, exists only for lung cancer, with respect to smoking. In varying proportions, improved detection and treatment are essential in control of most cancers. Individual behavior, of course, plays a major role in initiating the services required for prompt detection and appropriate therapy. But the efforts, successes, and failures of individuals to obtain the required services appear certain to be affected by factors outside individual control as well as by personal intelligence, knowledge, and motivation. A single decade of the late twentieth century brought substantial changes in these factors.

The Availability of Care

If most Americans in fact depend on currently available treatment to reduce the threat of cancer to their survival—personal behavior or medical breakthroughs offer only limited hope—attention must turn to their ability to obtain such care. Questions must be asked not only about the supply of basics, such as physicians, surgeons, and hospital rooms, but also about the availability of *appropriate* care—services that match the specific needs of individual patients at crucial junctures in their fight for survival. A review of the arrangements under which Americans obtain health care suggests that many fail to obtain such care. Recent history suggests that appropriate care is becoming less rather than more readily available to large numbers of Americans.

Before deciding whether appropriate care is available to persons with cancer—already diagnosed or not even yet suspected—we need to understand two factors that inhibit the use of health care even when it is physically available. The first factor is monetary cost. It is a truism that the more goods and services cost, the fewer of them people will consume. This is as true of visits to physicians and dentists, surgical operations, and stays in hospitals as it is of ice cream cones, automobiles, and applications to expensive colleges.

The predominance of payment for health care by insurance companies and government programs rather than by patients themselves during the post–World War II years hid the relationship between costs and utilization of health services. But a major study published by the Rand Corporation in the 1980s revealed several important facts. The greater the portion of physician and hospital costs patients paid out of their own pockets, the fewer physician visits they made and the fewer hospital stays they experienced. The necessity of paying even a small percentage of the bill significantly diminished the patient's utilization of these services. "Free" care, however, resulted in marked increases in utilization.[19] In some important instances, the barrier to health care presented by out-of-pocket payment was as strong for those who clearly needed the service as for those who did not. A team of physician experts reviewed hospital records to determine whether the admission of several hundred patients was really necessary on medical grounds. Their review indicated that "copayment"—that is, out-of-pocket payment by the patient for a portion of his or her health care costs—had no effect on whether a patient's admission was or was not appropriate.[20]

Nonmonetary cost is a second factor that often deters people from obtaining health care. Costs of this nature encompass various forms of inconvenience that people must undergo in the process of seeking care. The physical and mental effort required to see a health professional is one nonmonetary cost. Distance from an individual's home to his or her source of health care will deter utilization because of the time and effort required for transportation. In some instances, the care-seeker may have to convince a receptionist or nurse that an appointment is truly necessary. Such persuasion may require the potential patient to expend mental effort and undergo emotional discomfort. The most obvious nonmonetary cost is waiting: for a turn to speak with an office functionary to make an appointment; between the time the appointment is made and the actual visit with a physician or other health professional; at the doctor's office or clinic to be seen. Doubtlessly, innumerable would-be seekers of health care waiting "on hold" have decided that their problems were not sufficiently serious for medical attention, that they might delay awhile longer to see whether their symptoms abated, or that they were too fearful of what the physician might find to see the process through.

Nonmonetary costs of this kind are most frequent in situations where immediate monetary costs to the patient are absent or low. The visitor to a large, urban clinic serving the poor can count on needing to demonstrate the urgency of his or her condition and then waiting for access to the health professional. The long delays in scheduling of surgery or other specialty care in Britain's National Health Service are legendary. Patients do not pay directly for service in the British system, but receive care as a benefit funded by public taxation.

Mainstream Americans are most likely to encounter these nonmonetary costs in so-called health maintenance organizations (HMOs). Health care providers of this kind have existed in the United States since the 1920s, offering comprehensive physician services and hospitalization for a fixed, prepaid fee. Until the 1970s, providers of this kind were known simply as prepaid group practices or plans. The best known of these plans are the Kaiser Foundation Health Plan, the Health Insurance Plan of Greater New York (HIP), and Group Health Cooperative of Puget Sound. In 1971, a wary Nixon administration sponsored legislation to encourage the establishment of prepaid health care providers, coining the term *HMO* to popularize the program. But in the absence of convincing evidence that HMOs are particularly effective in preventing disease and maintaining health, most health care professionals understand the term to indicate plans in which the subscriber pays a fixed fee in advance for services. Such plans are distinguished from "fee-for-service" care, under which the recipient (or his or her insurance carrier) pays for each episode of utilization.

The frequently noted experience of waiting for care in organizations that do not levy major charges to patients for each episode of service may be explained as an economy measure. Providing health care is expensive, and providers must find ways to control utilization when direct charges are not imposed. HMOs save money by not carrying extra resources in the form of readily available physician appointment slots and hospital beds; these are unproductive when not in constant use. But patients may pay a price in the form of extra waiting time for these resources, and they may find access further restricted by the need of their doctors to rush through examinations and give rapid, sometimes incomprehensible, answers to their questions.

It seems unlikely that HMOs and other organizations that provide services without direct charges to their patients *intentionally* discourage necessary care—although some instances of this nature have been documented.[21] Indeed, the Rand study found that preventive visits were more frequent in an HMO than in community settings where patients made direct payments for service.[22] But the possibility that patients in some HMOs may not receive appropriate and timely care remains a topic of concern.

Future social historians may come to regard the mid-1970s as a kind of golden age, in which large numbers of Americans escaped significant out-of-pocket payment for their health care. In 1977, the federal government carried out a national study to determine how Americans paid for the health services they received. The study covered a representative sample of 14,000 households. It indicated that almost one-fourth of the United States population incurred no personal expenditures for health care in that year. Among those who visited a physician or dentist, obtained prescriptions for eyeglasses or medications, or spent time in a hospital, over half expended less than $100 out of pocket.[23]

Even during this era, however, most Americans had to rely on their personal incomes and savings for certain types of services. In 1977, over 150 million Americans under age sixty-five—about 80 percent of the individuals in this age group—were beneficiaries of private health insurance plans. Of these, almost 98 percent had coverage for stays in the hospital. The vast majority paid nothing for hospital room and board; over 70 percent received 100 percent coverage for a semiprivate hospital room. Insurance coverage was less generous for the charges of practitioners who treated patients in these hospital rooms. Almost all privately insured patients under age sixty-five in 1977 received benefits for surgeons' and physicians' fees for services delivered in the hospital; but only about 44 percent received benefits equal to the total of their surgeons' "usual, customary, and reasonable" fees, and only about 32 percent received reimbursement for all in-hospital physician charges.

Insurance coverage was still weaker for physician services outside the hospital. Only 83 percent of private insurance beneficiaries had coverage for office visits to physicians, and only 16 percent of these beneficiaries were covered for 100 percent of the usual, customary, and reasonable fees. Almost all privately insured patients (93 percent) had coverage for diagnostic tests in a physician's office, but over 60 percent were reimbursed for less than usual, reasonable, and customary charges or faced limits on the total amount they could recover for such procedures.[24]

Americans with private health insurance in the mid-1970s generally had little to fear about incurring major out-of-pocket expenses. Throughout the economically booming 1950s and 1960s, private insurance—typically provided by employers as fringe benefits to their employees—covered ever-increasing areas of need, from hospitalization to doctor visits to mental health. Occasionally, patients might receive bills for some services performed by a surgeon or an anesthesiologist. Most often, bills for uncovered expenses would come for visits to the physician's office, particularly if the doctor had ordered diagnostic tests. Out-of-pocket expenditures of this kind could be small compared with the uninsured portion of a surgeon's fee, but for most individuals and families they were much more frequent.

By the mid-1980s, many Americans with private health insurance found themselves with considerably poorer coverage. Faced with higher costs and increasing competition from abroad, businesses began paying closer attention to the costs of health care. These costs had been rising even more rapidly than those of other goods and services throughout the boom years, and were reflected in the premiums health insurance companies charged employers to insure their workers. Out-of-pocket payments increased in both frequency and magnitude for nearly all private health insurance beneficiaries. Premiums themselves increased, and many employers who had, in effect, paid these charges on behalf of their employees began requiring employees to pay at least part of their own premiums.

But in health insurance, the biggest news of the 1980s was copayment. This concept expresses the belief that individuals themselves should share the expenses for their health care with the third-party payer. Under copayment, both the insurance company and the beneficiary share liability for expenses that arise from the beneficiary's use of health services. In the beneficiary's day-to-day life, copayment takes the form of "deductibles" and "coinsurance." Deductibles require people to pay a fixed amount per unit of service (such as a physician visit or hospital stay) or period of time (typically one year) before the insurance company pays anything. Coinsurance means that beneficiaries must pay a percentage of the charges for each unit of service, whatever previous payments may have been.

Consultants and experts in health care "cost containment" have hailed deductibles and coinsurance as economy measures. But for the consumer, these developments often mean hefty financial obligations. Typically, insurance plans are structured to offer lower premiums in exchange for higher deductibles and coinsurance, motivating many beneficiaries to risk later liabilities in exchange for savings on the "front end." By the mid-1980s, it was not uncommon for a family to pay several thousand dollars in deductibles before its insurance plan covered *any* expenses. Typically, the privately insured individual received "80–20" coverage, the insurance plan paying 80 percent of charges (after deductibles) and the beneficiary responsible for the remaining 20 percent. Scope of coverage remained about the same as in the 1970s for visits to physicians and tests received in their offices. But direct responsibility for hospital care charges became a much greater likelihood for the insured individual. About 40 percent of U.S. employers paid all hospital room-and-board charges for their employees in 1986, whereas well over 80 percent of employers had paid these charges as recently as 1981.

Large numbers of Americans, of course, do not have private insurance coverage but receive their care under government programs. The largest of these is Medicare, a Social Security–based program intended to pay the health care costs of Americans over sixty-five years old and certain other groups. The Medicare program consists of Part A, which covers hospital costs, and Part B, which covers fees for physician services, diagnostic tests, and other outpatient services. Like private health insurance, Medicare requires deductibles and coinsurance. As with private plans, coverage is most complete for hospital charges and considerably less comprehensive for professional fees and outpatient diagnostic tests. Contrary to popular belief, Medicare paid less than 50 percent of costs incurred by its beneficiaries in the mid-1980s.

Elderly Americans typically limit their monetary risks by purchasing "medigap" policies from private insurance companies to supplement their Medicare benefits. About 65 percent of Medicare beneficiaries hold such policies. Most of these policies provide full coverage for inpatient charges not covered by Medicare, except for very long hospital stays. Like other forms of private health insurance, though, medigap policies usually provide considerably less extensive coverage for outpatient care. Only about one-third of Medicare beneficiaries have medigap policies that cover visits to a physician's office or outpatient diagnostic services.[25] A majority of elderly Americans, then, rely at least partially on income, savings, and other private resources for outpatient and diagnostic care.

By some measures, Medicare held up better than other forms of health insurance in the cost-conscious atmosphere of the 1980s. Between 1975 and 1982, the personal liability of Medicare beneficiaries for outpatient services declined from 71 to 52 percent of charges. But in this same period, the average annual liability increased from $151 to $344 per enrollee, as health care costs escalated.[26]

In the 1980s, older Americans were not economically disadvantaged as a group, thanks to a stable Social Security system and generous pensions provided by employers during the boom years. Health insurance available to truly poor people and the changes it has undergone are considerably more complex than for those eligible for Medicare. Poor people in the United States include many social categories: welfare recipients (principally beneficiaries of the Aid to Families of Dependent

Children program), the "working poor," transient adults, and undocumented aliens, to name the most obvious.

In the same year that Medicare was enacted, Congress passed legislation mandating the Medicaid program for the poor. Originally envisaged as a program offering comprehensive services to poor people, Medicaid is administered by individual states and paid for by monies from both the federal government and state treasuries. Since its enactment, Medicaid has proven considerably more costly than originally expected. Consequently, state governments have restricted eligibility to some favored categories of poor people—notably, those receiving cash assistance under existing public aid programs. While 92 percent of Americans with incomes below the official poverty level received benefits under Medicaid in 1977, this figure declined to 72 percent in 1982 and 64 percent in 1984.[27] Persons not qualified to receive Medicaid must look to a complex of public and private facilities offering care to the indigent. A growing number use clinics or emergency rooms based in large county hospitals as sources of last resort for health care.

The health maintenance organization (HMO)—which provides a broad range of services to its subscribers for a fixed, prepaid fee—has received considerable attention as a means of preserving access to care while restraining costs. Individuals often find such plans attractive because they charge lower rates and offer more comprehensive benefits than conventional health insurance. Businesses and public agencies, which often provide insurance for employees or program beneficiaries, have experimented widely with HMOs. Businesses often cover all payments for HMO membership for employees who elect to join; at least one major firm for a time required new employees to enroll. Federal legislation has encouraged Medicare beneficiaries to join HMOs. At least one state has experimented with establishing a special organization with characteristics highly similar to an HMO for Medicaid recipients.

Since the 1970s, HMO enrollment has grown as rapidly as copayment in conventional health insurance. Between 1980 and 1987, HMO enrollment virtually doubled, from 15 to 30 million Americans. In 1987, there were nearly 700 such plans functioning in the United States. This growth contrasts starkly with earlier days, when HMOs enrolled tiny minorities of the population. Growth has been most rapid among employed individuals who receive health insurance from their employers.

Many of today's HMOs, however, are different from those that characterized the industry prior to the 1970s. In the earlier era, HMOs

were typically nonprofit organizations owned by either private founda-
tions (such as Kaiser) or their members (such as Group Health Cooperative of Puget Sound). They were usually staffed by socially conscious,
nonconformist physicians whose entire practice took place within the
HMO. Local medical establishments distanced themselves from HMOs,
labeled them "socialized medicine," and ostracized their staffs. Today's
HMO is as likely to be an investor-owned, profit-seeking organization
as a nonprofit organization. For-profit firms, such as Maxicare and
Cigna, are now major operators in the HMO business. Most of the
recently formed HMOs write contracts with outside physician groups,
allowing individual practitioners to see non-HMO patients on a fee-for-
service basis and to contract as desired with other HMOs. The newer
HMOs typically employ aggressive marketing staffs, aiming recruitment
drives at young, relatively healthy populations least likely to consume
the organization's resources.

Both copayment and HMO enrollment may function as barriers to
health care utilization. Copayment represents monetary cost, which
elementary economics would suggest reduces consumption. HMOs are
believed by many to impose nonmonetary costs in the form of greater
levels of effort to obtain appointments with health professionals and
longer waits for services than are encountered in fee-for-service settings.

In the years when these innovations grew most rapidly, in fact, per
capita use of health services in the United States decreased. Some comparative findings from a recent UCLA study illustrate changes that
occurred in the 1980s. Between 1982 and 1986, Americans' overall use
of services (both physician visits and hospitalization) declined. The
percentage without a visit to a physician in the preceding year rose from
19 to 33; the percentage unable to identify a usual source of care rose
from 11 to 18. Use of hospital services declined more slowly than
physician visits—the percentage hospitalized in the past year falling
from 9 in 1982 to 7 in 1986. Especially striking was the finding that
many Americans did not seek medical care in response to apparent need.
The study indicated that one in six who had "an identifiable chronic and
serious illness (such as cancer, heart disease, diabetes, and stroke) did not
see a physician even once during the year."[28]

The "golden age" of health care in the United States—in which large
numbers of individuals enjoyed prompt access to the physician or hospital of their choice with low out-of-pocket payment—declined rapidly in
the 1980s, at least for individuals who depended on their employers to
supply health insurance coverage. Developments were more complex for

those who depended on the government to pay their health care bills. Programs that served the old, the disabled, and the poor of various descriptions fared unevenly in the atmosphere of growing fiscal constraint. The UCLA study reported a growing disparity in health care utilization by the poor and nonpoor between 1982 and 1986, a fact that signaled the reversal of a fifty-year trend toward equality. But in these years, more Americans in *all* walks of life began having to pay more and negotiate their way through an increasingly complicated maze of bureaucrats in order to see the doctor. These developments have raised questions about access to care for conditions from the most minor to the most immediately life-threatening.

Personal Choice and Avoidable Mortality

In the closing years of the twentieth century, obtaining appropriate care for any illness became more difficult for most Americans. The individual's knowledge of the health care system and how to use it to meet his or her own needs became especially important under these conditions. No "patient advocate" will ever replace the individual's responsibility for taking the steps necessary to maintain health and prolong life. An understanding of the factors that lead to survival from cancer, such as those described in the following chapters, enables the individual to use an increasingly complex and expensive health care system to his or her best advantage. Signs have started to appear that America faces an increasing problem of "avoidable mortality" in cancer—deaths that are *preventable* through appropriate use of medical treatment available today. People as individuals must take the initiative to ensure that they and their loved ones do not become included among these unfortunate cases.

Even the best-informed and most well-to-do citizens obtain their health care under conditions not of their own making. Changes in health insurance and the establishment of HMOs come about through decisions of business leaders, public officials, union negotiators, benefits managers, and other representatives of interest groups seeking ways to live with the rising cost of health care. Since the availability of health care depends strongly on government or corporate policy, it is surprising that health care delivery only intermittently becomes a visible major public issue. Health issues outside familiar areas such as toxic waste typically receive little attention in public discussion. Health care was a major election issue in the early 1970s, when concern for the disadvantaged and proposals for national health insurance made headlines. Although individual Americans may have become increasingly concerned about their health care benefits, however, elections in the 1980s highlighted other issues.

Our individualistic political culture may explain this lack of major attention to health care in public discourse. When free from serious illness, most Americans think of themselves as self-reliant and fully responsible for their own health and well-being. In this perspective, survival of the threat posed by cancer depends on individual actions such as avoidance of cancer hazards, awareness of "warning signs" that may reveal occurrence of early cancer, or willingness to make appointments with physicians in response to such signs or on a precautionary basis. Outlook on life, the "willingness to fight," and other positive features of individual character are widely believed to be effective in an individual's efforts to survive cancer.

No matter how self-reliant Americans may consider themselves, however, the social groupings they belong to and the resources they command will influence their behavior. Researchers have identified a variety of distinct features of the individual's background and environment that affect his or her seeking of health care. Steven Shortell, a leading investigator in this area, has summarized the factors that will prompt an individual to seek care, to delay contacting a physician, and to request episodic treatment or continuing care.[29] A well-known model focuses on three factors—"predisposing," "enabling," and "perceived medical need"—that explain the seeking of care. Shortell explains:

Predisposing variables include age, sex, marital status, family size, ethnicity, personal beliefs about health services, and attitudes toward physicians. Enabling variables include family income, insurance coverage, the availability of a regular source of care, and facility and provider per capita ratios. Medical need variables include disability days, symptoms, perceived health status, and physician-evaluated severity of the diagnosis and symptoms.

Research in the tendency of individuals to seek health care for either diagnosis or treatment recognizes that a combination of factors explains individual actions. Thus, a young, well-educated woman may be "predisposed" to obtaining regular Pap screening, but the supply of gynecologists in her locale, an "enabling" factor, may be too low to allow her to obtain the service without delay. The monetary and nonmonetary costs of health services discussed above are enabling factors. All factors in the model are nonbiomedical. The "medical need" variable, for instance, is nonbiomedical because it reflects the individual's *perception* of his or her condition.

The government is becoming more aware of the importance of these factors and the need to formulate effective responses. Consequently, since the mid-1960s, the National Cancer Institute—the largest single research organization in the United States and an agency of the federal Department of Health and Human Services—has conducted a "cancer control" program. As it has monitored cancer death rates, this agency has become increasingly concerned with the avoidable-mortality problem. In a report citing 143 studies and documents, officials of the National Cancer Institute identified a wide variety of "social barriers" to cancer detection and therapy.[30] Cultural factors appear crucial to these officials. Cervical cancer provides a useful illustration of cultural and personal barriers because of its involvement with a sex organ. A compelling line of thought favors development of outreach programs (such as mobile Pap smear screening in the community) carried out by "indigenous health workers" to help overcome class suspicions and cultural barriers. Responding to such concerns, the National Cancer Institute and the American Cancer Society have set scientists to the task of learning more about cultural barriers to health screening, particularly in the Hispanic and Asian communities, and developing effective interventions.

Most of the research that scientists have conducted thus far has concentrated on the individual's perception of health care, evaluation of its efficacy, and motivation to use it. Many social factors are considered, but these are tied closely to the individual's cultural background or personal attributes (such as sex and age) that may affect his or her predisposition to seek health care. Public and workplace-based cancer programs typically confine themselves to this approach. These factors are important. But quite apart from culture and personality, the need for individuals to pay for their health care and negotiate an increasingly complicated system of specialists and hospitals seems likely to increase mortality that, from a biomedical point of view, can be prevented. Comparative figures presented at the beginning of this chapter indicate that death rates for some cancers dropped swiftly for the disadvantaged in the 1960s and 1970s. These were years when, because of the inception and expansion of government programs, health care became more accessible than ever to the poor and elderly. Those concerned with the problems of the poor must ask serious questions about diminishing support in this area.

But these factors affect nonpoor people as well. As discussed above, even working people with private health insurance plans receive relatively scanty coverage for diagnostic services. Because these services are particularly important for early detection, their underutilization may increase the risk of dying from cancer for many relatively advantaged people. A recent report on mammography for detection of breast cancer illustrates this point. The American Cancer Society recommends a baseline mammogram, a highly effective X-ray method for detecting early tumors, for women thirty-five through thirty-nine, and then one every year or two for women over forty. Some reports indicate that mammography may reduce the mortality rate from breast cancer by 30 percent. But specialists say that only 13 percent of women at risk are now being screened. A major reason is that screening is not usually covered by insurance. As late as 1985, major insurance companies—Aetna, Prudential, and the Blue Cross and Blue Shield Association—did not cover routine screening examinations. The absence of such coverage means that patients must pay out of pocket for such proven early-detection procedures as mammography and Pap tests.[31] While the cost of a Pap test was less than $10 in the mid-1980s, that of mammography screening was between $100 and $150—enough to make many a working woman hesitate to make it a regular part of her health care program.

If anything, health care benefits are being reduced faster for working people who obtain insurance through their employers than for the disadvantaged who receive health care under government funding. Nobody knows the effects these reductions will have on health and life expectancy. Changes in cancer survival rates may emerge as the earliest visible outcomes.

◆   ◆   ◆   ◆   ◆

True victory over cancer probably will not come in this generation, or even the next. If previous patterns continue, medical research will not produce breakthroughs of a sufficient magnitude to reduce the overall threat. Personal avoidance of cancer hazards, though important, will provide individuals with only partial protection. It is doubtful that all known environmental and behavioral factors associated with cancer produce even half of the malignancies that occur every year in the United States.

In view of the prevalence of cancer and the threat it represents to the length and quality of life, all means known to be effective in promoting survival must be utilized. The following chapters aim at achieving a better understanding of the nonbiomedical factors associated with cancer survival. An understanding of the relative importance of social, psychological, financial, individual, and health care system–related factors can serve as the basis for better-informed individual strategies for avoiding cancer and obtaining favorable outcomes in treatment.

Beyond personal interests, however, a better understanding of "who survives cancer" underscores the importance of broader issues for the century to come. Do we desire a society where people must be outstandingly clever or well-off to survive? Do we believe that only the exceptional should benefit from the best achievements of modern technology? To what extent do we believe in sacrificing individual choice and life chances for the good of the whole? A greater appreciation of these issues may help strengthen the position of health care as a key item on the public agenda. This inquiry requires, first, an overview of the "cancer problem" as it existed in the late twentieth century and an understanding of what is meant by "survival." Unusual features distinguish cancer from other diseases. This overview helps define appropriate goals for medical and individual action.

CHAPTER TWO

The Disease and Its Survivors

The twentieth century saw humankind all but bring the globe under push-button control. Conquests over illness ranked among the century's greatest achievements. The richer nations came close to ridding themselves of deadly infectious diseases; maladies such as smallpox and plague, which had terrified humankind from its earliest days, were virtually eradicated worldwide. But science did not succeed in "conquering" cancer. As the century drew to a close, technology available to fight malignant disease still seemed primitive when compared with that of computers, telecommunications, and air travel. The century's advances in medical technology did include some important benefits for those who contracted cancer. But large gaps and considerable uncertainty remained in the effectiveness of cancer treatment. In the absence of reliable and cheap cures, cancer remained a major threat to longevity and the quality of life.

Humankind remained unable to dispose of cancer despite the application of considerable intelligence, inventiveness, and effort. The nature of cancer as an illness has raised an unprecedented challenge for doctors and scientists. Like many "modern" diseases, cancer differs markedly from the illnesses that usually claimed the lives of our forebears. The term *cancer* encompasses hundreds of different diseases. A single case of cancer may be vexingly complex. Attempts at cure may require a multiplicity of different treatments, whose sequence must be calibrated to the specific characteristics of each individual case. Today's cancer specialists fight the disease with techniques much more varied and complex than the pills, shots, and operations used against strep throat, syphilis, and gallstones. But they face much more recalcitrant adversaries.

An understanding of the factors that determine cancer survival must begin with basic facts and perspectives provided by the traditional health sciences. This chapter, as well as Chapters 3 and 4, draws on these disciplines. Traditional health sciences, such as medicine, genetics, and molecular biology, provide an understanding of the biological features of cancer and its treatment. Without this information, a search for other factors that may affect cancer survival would be meaningless. Furthermore, examination of research and practice in the health sciences helps delineate the extent of their contributions to cancer survival. An understanding of the limitations of medicine and biomedical research underscores the importance of human behavior and the organization and delivery of care in preventing biologically unnecessary deaths.

This chapter draws on biomedical science to delineate the features of cancer that distinguish it from other diseases and, at the same time, make it virtually impossible to comprehend as a single disease itself. The chapter looks to public health for a basic epidemiology of cancer, its prevalence, and the distribution of its many forms throughout the population. It borrows from the thinking of biostatisticians to identify appropriate concepts of cancer survival, which, like the biological features of the disease itself, are complex and differ in applicability from case to case.

Cancer: A Complex Phenomenon

Perhaps more than any other illness, "cancer" does not constitute a monolithic threat to life. A summary of both the features that all cancers have in common and the major variations in the disease provides key information related to several basic questions: Which individuals are most likely to contract the disease? Why are some forms of cancer highly curable and others especially lethal? What are the most realistic goals in treatment? How should doctors and patients evaluate options for cure?

THE NATURE OF MALIGNANT DISEASE

All cancers begin as single cells somewhere in the body. Every component of the body—bones, muscles, blood, glands, the linings of tubes and ducts—consists of microscopic cells. Most cells periodically reproduce by splitting in half, creating two daughter cells identical with the original. The additional cells replace those that have been damaged or died. A cancer begins when the original cell loses its capacity to pass on normal characteristics because the DNA, vital in the process of replication, is damaged or functions improperly. The abnormal cells resulting from this process then reproduce, giving rise to larger and larger numbers of aberrant cells. Generally, cancer cells reproduce more rapidly than normal ones. In time, the resulting cell mass or tumor tends to invade adjacent tissues and organs. In the process called *metastasis,* individual cells break off from the original mass, circulate through the body in the bloodstream or lymph system, seed in far-flung organs and tissues, and give rise to new tumors.

Cancer cells and tumors harm the organism because they serve no useful physiological purpose and interfere with or destroy the functioning of healthy tissues and organs. Lung cancer illustrates several typical disease syndromes. As tumors develop in locations near their origins, they cause symptoms by compressing the air passages within the lung. The resulting obstructions cause coughing, spitting up of blood, and reduction of oxygen in the bloodstream. As the tumor becomes larger or spreads to nearby organs, it may obstruct important blood vessels or weaken bones. When distant metastases occur—as is frequent in lung cancer—tumors may appear in vital organs such as the brain or liver. Death may take place when these distant organs no longer function adequately—for example, when an involved part of the brain can no longer control an important body function.

Cancers also cause sickness and death by less direct means: they may leave basic organ functions intact, but cause death from general debilitation. For reasons that scientists do not yet understand, many forms of cancer reduce the body's ability to fight infection. Many people with cancers other than lung, for example, die of pneumonia. The spreading of cancer to the bones weakens the patient's ability to support body weight and increases the likelihood of fracture. Cancers that begin in the prostate gland may, for example, spread to the pelvis or spine, resulting in fractures whose crippling effects hasten death. Some cancers and cancer therapies make it difficult for patients to eat and drink, increasing the risk of mortality due to inadequate nutrition or dehydration.

The diagnosis of a malignancy is usually experienced as a sudden, shocking event, precipitating both the patient and the physician into intense activity aimed at control or cure. But the development of cancer typically mirrors that of other life-threatening diseases, such as heart disease, stroke, and emphysema. These diseases, which are widespread in modern society, differ from those that swept earlier civilizations, infecting vast numbers of people rapidly and killing many in short order. Like heart disease, stroke, and emphysema, cancer is usually a *chronic* illness, developing in definite steps over a period that may last many years before becoming an obvious illness and threatening the patient's life.

Most laypeople are well aware that cancer develops in *stages*. Physicians use many different schemes, often tailored to the specifics of different forms of the disease, to denote the stages of cancer. All these schemes have the basic characteristic of distinguishing the degree to which the cancer has become disseminated throughout the body. A summary of a variety of schemes for staging lung cancer illustrates the logic of such classifications:

> *Stage I (localized)*. Microscopic examination of cells from a tumor reveals cancer. Generally, the tumor must be small and not have extended to structures contiguous with the lung, such as the chest wall. Cancer cells must be absent in all lymph nodes.
>
> *Stage II (regional spread)*. The tumor must be larger (greater than 3 centimeters). Cancer cells must be found in nearby lymph nodes, but the disease cannot have spread to other organs or lymph nodes beyond the immediate area.
>
> *Stage III (distant spread)*. The tumor itself is usually large, has extended to the chest wall or diaphragm, or causes highly visible fluid secretion or obstructed breathing; cancer cells have spread at least as far as the lymph nodes around the windpipe; tumors have appeared in distant organs, such as the brain and liver.

Less familiar but of equal importance are a number of steps that occur in the development of cancer *before* the appearance of an actual lesion.[1] The first step is known as *initiation*. A malfunction in the reproductive biochemistry in a single, normal cell causes a few atypical cells to come into being. These cells have no immediate tendency to become active cancers; they lie dormant rather than reproducing rapidly or invading other tissues. Their presence produces no visible signs unless a second step, *promotion*, occurs. In this step, conditions favorable to the growth of the original cell population come into existence, giving rise to visible masses that are immediately cancerous or start as benign and become malignant. Even an early-stage cancer producing a few faint symptoms, then, may represent a relatively late phase in the development of a malignancy. In some cancers, the latent period, between initiation and appearance of symptoms, has been estimated to last between thirty and forty years.

DIFFERENCES AMONG MALIGNANCIES

For individuals and professionals concerned with promoting survival, the variations among individual forms of malignant disease are crucial. In general, it is virtually meaningless to ask whether cancer is "curable" or how long a cancer patient may be expected to live. The answer to either question depends largely on three factors: the *anatomical site* at which the cancer originates, the *stage* at which it is diagnosed, and the *histology,* or specific type of cell of which it is composed.

Figures 1 through 3 summarize the "cancer problem" as it played out in the United States in 1990. In that year, the American Cancer Society estimated that 1,040,000 Americans would be diagnosed with cancer, and 510,000 would die of the disease.[2] These figures do not mean that nearly half of those who were diagnosed in 1990 would die in that year. Most of these deaths would occur among people diagnosed in earlier years.

Figure 1 indicates the most frequent cancers that experts expected to occur in the United States in 1990. The figure provides information on the "incidence" of each form of cancer for 1990; that is, the number of new cases diagnosed in that year. It presents the number of new cases of cancer at each "primary site," or the location in the body where it first appeared. The figure provides separate totals for men and women. It includes data on only one form of skin cancer, malignant melanoma. While other forms of skin cancer were expected to number 600,000 in 1990, these spread very slowly if at all and seldom cause death.

The nine separate forms of cancer represented in Figure 1 encompass almost 75 percent of the new malignancies expected in the United States in 1990. Not represented in the figure are many less frequent but hardly rare forms of cancer, such as pancreatic (29,000 cases expected in 1990), stomach (23,000 cases), and liver (15,000 cases). It is important to remember that the majority of Americans with cancer in 1990 had contracted the disease in previous years. The total "prevalence" of cancer in 1990—that is, the number of individuals with cancer (including those permanently cured)—was around 6,000,000.[3]

An overview of survival rates for the most common forms of cancer reveals great variability by site. Figure 2 summarizes the survivability of

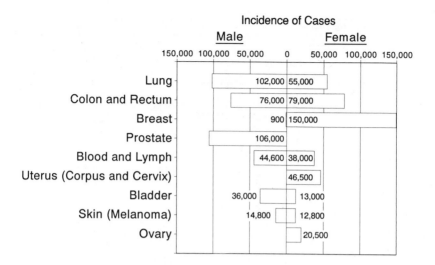

Fig. 1. *Cancers diagnosed, by sex and most frequent site, 1990. Source:* Cancer Facts and Figures 1990. *Atlanta: American Cancer Society, 1990.*

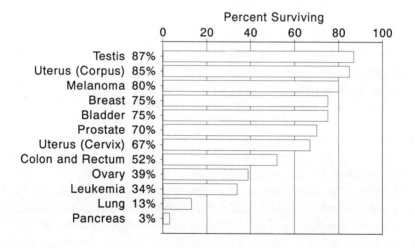

Fig. 2. *Five-year survival rates by most frequent cancer site, 1990. Source:* Cancer Facts and Figures 1990. *Atlanta: American Cancer Society, 1990.*

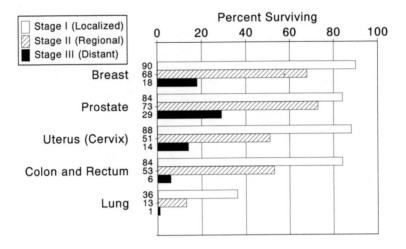

Fig. 3. *Five-year survival rates by cancer stage: differences by site. Source:* Cancer Facts and Figures 1990. *Atlanta: American Cancer Society, 1990.*

twelve cancers in the United States based on records compiled between 1974 and 1985. The primary site of the cancer made an overwhelming difference in chance for survival. Figure 2 indicates the percentage of individuals who survived five years or more after diagnosis, a widely used benchmark to signify successful treatment. For all stages combined, highs of 87 and 85 percent survived five years or more for cancers of the testis and uterine corpus; lows of 13 and 3 percent survived a similar length of time for cancers of the lung and pancreas.

Stage makes a statistical difference in survival of most if not all the forms of cancer. Figure 3 lists five-year survival rates by stage for the most frequently diagnosed cancers in 1990. For all diseases represented in Figure 3, persons diagnosed in Stage I had a considerably greater likelihood of surviving five years than those diagnosed in Stage III. Among patients with lung cancer, for example, those diagnosed in Stage I had a thirty-five times greater chance of surviving five years than those diagnosed in Stage III.

But early-stage diagnosis does not always increase survival chances in a meaningful way. For some cancers, diagnosis is almost never made in the early stage. Lung cancer is a telling example. In one study, which omitted the most aggressive form of the disease and meticulously confirmed degree of dissemination, fewer than 18 percent of the cases were diagnosed in Stage I.[4] In other cancers, people may have a *relative* advantage from early-stage diagnosis but still stand only a small chance of long-term survival. Even at Stage I, for example, only 6 percent of patients with pancreatic cancer survive five years.[5]

Figure 3 actually represents the variability of cancer survival in a highly simplified fashion. A major study by the National Cancer Institute, based on over 500,000 Americans diagnosed with cancer between 1973 and 1977, identified 304 different primary sites.[6] Physicians and scientists draw important distinctions within the individual cancer sites listed in Figure 1. Thus, colon cancer may occur in a particular segment of the large intestine, so that the patient may have a cancer of the sigmoid colon, descending colon, transverse colon, ascending colon, or cecum. These four, moreover, include only the most common forms of colon cancer.

In addition, major differences occur among cancers according to the microscopic characteristics of the cancer cells themselves, or "histology." The National Cancer Institute report identified up to twenty specific histological types associated with some anatomical sites. In lung cancer, for instance, the tumors may be designated as squamous cell carcinomas, small or oat cell carcinomas, or adenocarcinomas, to name the most frequently diagnosed; there are also rarer, exotically named tumors such as giant or spindle cell carcinomas, clear cell adenocarcinomas, or signet ring cell carcinomas.

Although histology is a characteristic of cancer less familiar to most people than site or stage, it is often an important clue to prognosis. Summarizing studies of patients who had received surgery for lung cancer before 1982, one authority reported strikingly different five-year survival rates for different histological types: bronchoalveolar carcinoma, 51 percent; squamous cell carcinoma, 33 percent; adenocarcinoma, 26 percent; small cell carcinoma, 1 percent.[7] All forms of lung cancer are serious. When all stages and histologies are analyzed together, only 13 percent of those diagnosed with this disease are found to live five years or more. Patients with some forms of lung cancer, however, have significant chances for survival if diagnosed and treated early. In other forms—most notably, lung cancer of the small cell type—stage apparently makes little difference. This histological type of lung cancer has been characterized as "explosively" metastatic, forming multiple lesions in the lung and other organs before it produces symptoms or becomes detectable.

Other features of individual cells may distinguish cancers of the same anatomical site. *Grade,* for example, refers to the differentiation among cells as they appear under a microscope. "Well-differentiated" cells bear close resemblance to normal ones; they are relatively uniform in size and have clearly defined features, such as nuclei and boundaries. "Poorly differentiated" cells vary significantly in size and shape and have less well-defined features. Poor differentiation may, as in cancer of the prostate, indicate a poorer chance of survival. In some cancers, cells become less and less well differentiated as the disease develops. Cells in apparently similar cancers may differ in their ability to bind with certain hormones. These differences may, in turn, affect a patient's treatment options and life expectancy.

Possible combinations of site and histology run into the thousands. In some ways, each site-histology combination represents a different disease. Some cancers remain localized, while others move aggressively to invade nearby organs or metastasize to distant sites. Some forms of cancer spread beyond their points of origin in regular, predictable ways, spawning metastatic lesions in the same organs in nearly every case; others are more nearly random in the speed and pattern by which they spread. Each site-histology combination presents unique problems for the physician in planning treatment.

Site, stage, and histology answer a large part of the question "Who survives cancer?" People who develop cancers with especially bad combinations of these disease features have virtually no chance of living more than a few years; those with more favorable forms of the disease may have excellent chances for long-term survival. At least in the late twentieth century, these basic biological features acted as boundaries to the benefits of medicine.

The "Cure" for Cancer: Defining an Elusive Goal

Cancer differs markedly from diseases that predominated in the early 1900s. Many of these diseases, such as diphtheria or cholera, were *acute* in nature, striking suddenly and doing their damage fast. Prevention and cure required simple, definitive, and rapidly administered interventions. By contrast, cancer often develops slowly and allows the patient to survive for many years. Of great importance is the fact that cancer is not really one disease but a very large *category* of diseases affecting many organs and systems. Medicine can be truly beneficial only if patients and physicians acknowledge these facts in setting goals. Science and public policy can ask appropriate questions only by acknowledging these realities. The biological features of cancer make "cure" and "survival," basic concerns of research and medicine, much more complex than they have traditionally been.

In comparison with treatment goals for other diseases, the goals of cancer treatment are difficult to define. Through most of the twentieth century, "cure" in the traditional sense was simply unavailable for many forms of cancer. Nevertheless, medicine offered significant benefits to cancer patients, including many of those with "incurable" diseases. For a majority of cancer patients, physicians possessed techniques that could prolong life and enhance function and comfort. As the century drew to a close, technology began to blur the distinction between arresting a malignancy and palliating its effects. Settling on firm criteria for success in cancer treatment became increasingly difficult. Still, scientists and citizens alike required and will continue to require such criteria to evaluate the benefits of treatment innovations—as well as the impacts of changes in methods and resources for delivering health care.

The traditional concept of cure—permanent removal of a disease—is often not an appropriate goal even in "treatable" malignancies. Traditional thinking about curing disease works well for acute illnesses, especially those that are infectious in nature. A man with an infected wound takes an antibiotic; swelling and pain recede, and normal color returns; in a few days, the man is "cured." Disappearance of signs of illness is the key. But in a person under treatment for cancer, removal of apparent signs of disease does not equal cure. In time, cancer often recurs after a tumor is excised, malignant cells having remained at the site of the original lesion or lodged undetected elsewhere in the body. It is quite often more accurate to characterize a successfully treated patient as having "no evidence of disease" or "in remission" rather than "cured."

In the absence of sure clinical indications of cure, many scientists use statistical definitions based on survival after diagnosis. "Five-year survival," for example, is often taken as an indication of cure, and is probably the most familiar of the criteria used. The comparative figures presented above use this criterion. Many interpret five-year survival to mean that a person who has experienced no recurrence for five years after initial treatment harbors no malignant cells or undetected tumors. After five years, it is assumed that he or she has no more likelihood of contracting cancer than anyone else, and that his or her life expectancy equals that of any other person with similar demographic characteristics.

This interpretation of five-year survival is faulty for many forms of cancer. Five-year survival is always a hopeful sign. But in general, people who have a history of cancer are more likely to develop malignancies in the future than people with no such history. Breast cancer is a frequently cited example of the limits of five-year survival as a definition of cure. In this disease, recurrences are known to take place in persons who evidence no signs of cancer ten or fifteen years after initial treatment. Prostatic cancer reveals another limitation of this often-cited criterion. A high proportion of men with this disease, which often develops very slowly, live for five years or more *even in the absence of treatment*. A Veterans Administration study of men with early-stage prostatic cancer showed that half of those who received no treatment whatsoever survived over seven years.[8] Still, many men eventually die of cancer of the prostate.

The five-year milestone, however, is quite meaningful in other forms of cancer. Some are curable in the traditional sense—namely, that all apparent evidence of disease is gone and recurrence unlikely. In these cancers, most deaths or signs of treatment failure occur within a few years of diagnosis. Five-year survival is clearly meaningful in colon and certain forms of lung cancer. A Norwegian study of several malignancies found that 70 percent of women who contracted colon cancer had life expectancies considerably lower than women of similar ages in the general population. In this group, half the women were found to have died within eight months. The remaining 30 percent, however, fell into a group with the same life expectancy as that of the general population of similarly aged women. Within this group, half the women survived thirteen years or more—the same survival picture as that of Norwegian women in similar age groups. Women who remained alive by the five-year mark could be counted among those with normal life expectancies.[9] Five-year survival is also a meaningful touchstone for cure for some lung cancer patients. As discussed in the preceding section, lung cancer may take several forms according to *histology*, the type of cell found to compose the tumor. People with small cell lung cancer almost never survive five years. But a significant percentage of those with other forms of lung cancer diagnosed and treated in early stage do survive many months thereafter. Those who survive to the five-year milestone have a life expectancy approximating that of similarly aged people in the general population.[10]

Prostate cancer serves as a contrasting example. The Norwegian study found that, among men with prostatic cancer, half died within three years of diagnosis. At the time of the study, half the men in similar age groups in the general population could be expected to live eight years or more. The prostatic cancer patients who survived five years still had life expectancies well below those in the normal population.[11]

This detailed examination suggests that *cure* is more likely in colon cancer and some forms of lung cancer than in malignancies of the prostate. In prostate cancer, life expectancy never reverts to normal. This observation seems paradoxical, in that both lung and colon cancer (at least in the United States) have lower five-year survival rates than prostatic cancer. In the Norwegian study, in fact, a higher percentage of men with prostatic cancer survived for five years than women with colon cancer. The difference in biological characteristics between colon and prostatic cancer helps explain this paradox. Prostatic cancer normally spreads slowly and causes death many years after it originates if other diseases do not intervene. Yet this disease is stubborn and often recurs after treatment. Colon cancer spreads more rapidly but may be removed more surely by timely surgery. A strong irony arises in comparison of the two diseases. The colon cancer patient is more often definitively cured. But the prostate cancer patient is more likely to survive five years or longer. According to many physicians, medical care is more beneficial to people with cancer of the colon. But nature is, in a sense, kinder to those with cancer of the prostate.

Evaluating survival chances, then, requires information in addition to the five-year survival rate. The "life table" is a useful alternative for comparing survival among cancer patients with different personal characteristics or receiving different treatments. Traditionally, insurance actuaries determine appropriate premiums for life insurance by constructing life tables that estimate an individual's chance of surviving through a given time interval. When used in the study of cancer survival, a life table can indicate the likelihood that an individual will survive to any point in time following his or her diagnosis—one month, six months, one year, five years, ten years. Scientists often draw graphs to show the average chance people in a study have of remaining alive at each successive milestone.

Life tables provide much more information on an individual's chances for life extension than five-year survival. An examination of a "survival curve" prepared from a life table of lung cancer patients (see Figure 4) illustrates this fact. The five-year survival rate for lung cancer in the middle to late twentieth century was an extremely dismal 13 percent. Even when the most dangerous form of lung cancer, small cell carcinoma, was excluded, only about one-third of the patients survived past

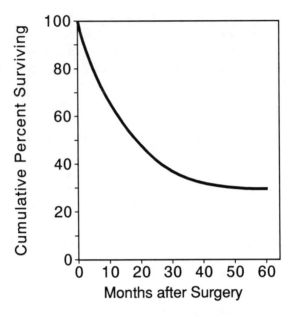

Fig. 4. *Survival of non–small cell lung cancer patients, stage II only. Abstracted from C.F. Mountain, "Assessment of the Role of Surgery for Control of Lung Cancer,"* Annals of Thoracic Surgery 24 (1977): 365–73.

the five-year mark. Yet for some people with lung cancer, Figure 4 provides encouragement.

Figure 4 indicates the percentages of people who remained alive at successive points in time following surgery for Stage II lung cancer. Those with the small cell type were excluded from the computations. The percentages of patients surviving decreased steadily until, about forty months after surgery, only about one-third of the patients remained alive by the five-year mark. But between the fourth and fifth year, the curve flattens. This flattening indicates that the percentage surviving remained constant—no more patients died. The survival curve, then, indicates that only a minority of lung cancer patients survive five years or more; but it also shows that those who survive to the five-year mark face risks of death comparable only to people of their own age with no cancer history. In all likelihood, these patients have been genuinely cured.

A survival curve for colon cancer in the Norwegian study would look similar to Figure 4, the percentage surviving becoming more or less constant after five years. But the survival curve for prostate or small cell lung cancer would never flatten out. A greater percentage of patients would have died at each successive time point.

Life tables and survival curves are particularly important in assessing treatment success in cancers where few patients survive five years or where, although life expectancy is long, true cure is uncertain. On the basis of life tables, scientists can determine the "relative risk" of death in one group as compared with another over a specific length of time. A statistic called a "risk ratio" is computed on the basis of the survival curves for both groups. If members of one group had a greater chance of dying in a given time period than members of another, their group's risk ratio would be greater than 1.

Scientists assessing alternative treatments for especially lethal cancers would base their analyses on life tables and risk ratios rather than on five-year survival. In instances where five-year or even one-year survival is infrequent, extension of life may still be desirable. The finding that a group of patients had a lower risk of dying than a group receiving a different form of care would signify successful therapy, worthy of being emulated in treatment of all patients. Five-year survival does not distinguish those treated more successfully; most if not all patients would have died by that time. But comparison of survival curves and risk ratios allows the distinction to be made.

Beyond Science: The Quality of Life

The quality of life constitutes still another perspective that must be considered in the assessment of survival. Like most chronic diseases, cancer may not only threaten survival but limit activity and the enjoyment of life. Pain, mood, and function have received considerable attention from scientists who assess the impact of cancer.[12] Scientists may objectively measure the degree of pain a patient experiences, the anxiety or depression he or she feels, or the difficulties in walking, eating, and communicating he or she encounters. But criteria for deciding when a disease makes life no longer "worth living" are ultimately individual and subjective.

These considerations raise important questions about the limits of science, technology, and medicine. In planning and assessing treatment, cancer patients and those who care for them often weigh perceived quality against prolongation of life. Palliative care, which emphasizes comfort—for example, reduction of pain—over extension of life, is an acceptable medical option. During the 1980s, following the hospice movement in England, hospitals and health care systems in the United

States established facilities designed to enable patients with advanced cancer to live comfortable, relatively normal lives during their last weeks. In the late twentieth century, both patients and physicians began to feel freer about alternative approaches to disease, and to accept death as a reasonable choice.

It seems likely that some people have always chosen to forgo available treatment that, while possibly extending life, probably would cause great physical discomfort and would not restore the vigor and mobility they enjoyed before becoming ill. But in the late twentieth century, such choices moved onto center stage in ethical and legal controversy. A movement arose in which patients signed "living wills," legal documents to limit the extent of care they desired when their conditions became biologically irreversible. Euthanasia, a practice alleged to have taken place informally and in secret for many years, burst into the public consciousness through a young physician's anonymous letter to one of the nation's top medical journals. In this letter, the physician revealed his thoughts and actions in a midnight encounter with "Debbie," a young woman dying of cancer:

> The room seemed filled with the patient's desperate effort to survive. Her eyes were hollow, and she had suprasternal and intercostal retractions with her rapid inspirations. She had not eaten or slept in two days. She had not responded to chemotherapy and was being given supportive care only. It was a gallows scene, a cruel mockery of her youth and unfulfilled potential. Her only words were, "Let's get this over with."
> I retreated with my thoughts to the nurses' station. The patient was tired and needed rest. I could not give her health but I could give her rest. I asked the nurse to draw 20 ml morphine sulfate into a syringe. Enough, I thought, to do the job. I took the syringe into the room and [said] I was going to give Debbie something that would let her rest and say goodbye. Debbie looked at the syringe, then laid her head on the pillow with her eyes open, watching what was left of the world. I injected the morphine intravenously and watched to see if my calculations on its effects would be correct. Within seconds her breathing slowed to a normal rate, her eyes closed, and her features softened as she seemed restful at last. . . . I waited for the inevitable next effect, depressing the respiratory drive. With clocklike certainty, within four minutes the breathing rate slowed even more, then became irregular, then ceased . . .
> It's over, Debbie.[13]

Whatever statistics and graphs scientists may formulate, simple extension of life cannot be the only consideration in the assessment of survival.

♦   ♦   ♦   ♦   ♦

The biology of cancer makes analysis of survival a complicated endeavor. At all times, it is important to remember that "cancer" constitutes a wide variety of diseases, many with very different characteristics and life expectancies. "Cure," moreover, is not an obvious goal. A truly meaningful analysis of treatment and other factors affecting cancer survival requires balancing several indicators of life extension, as well as considerations about survival entirely beyond science and statistics.

Despite the very real limitations of biological survival as a goal in cancer treatment, this book emphasizes the importance of factors that promote extension of life. It assumes that nearly everyone fights for life, and chooses to abandon the struggle only when disease has become truly unbearable and quality of life has gone into irreversible decline. Numerically expressed concepts of life extension, such as five-year survival and reduced relative risk, then, reflect valuable goals even with respect to patients who are ultimately terminal—as, indeed, are all mortals.

The "right to choose" has become a major cause among patient advocates. This position is defined most vocally with respect to terminal patients. But most cancer patients are not "terminal," if this is taken to mean that attempts at even limited extension of life are unlikely to succeed. During the months and years following diagnosis, most face periodic choices about treatment: What should it include? How extensive should it be? Where should it be received? The patient's hopes rest on these choices. For many, selecting the most appropriate options determines survival chances and the quality of life. To understand who is most likely to survive and how realities outside the arena of biological functioning affect survival, one must understand cancer treatment itself.

CHAPTER THREE

Cancer Treatment:
The Industry of Hope

Searching and hope dominate the lives of many cancer patients. In the knowledge of approaching death, people with advanced cancer may knock on many doors, hoping for a scientific breakthrough or miracle cure to save them. Journeys by twentieth-century cancer patients to the Mayo Clinic or Memorial Sloan-Kettering recall the pilgrimages to Lourdes and other spiritual healing centers of earlier days. To many, the vast industry that is modern health care must appear to harbor endless possibilities and options for cures. Today's miracle-seeker may apply at the research laboratory, the "alternative" practitioner's office, or both. Referrals from community physicians to major cancer centers are commonplace. Patients themselves may resort not just to one unproven cancer remedy but to sequences of such nostrums. The recollections of author John Gunther embody the behavior of the cure-seeker in its most energetic and eclectic form. Attempting to rescue their son from incurable brain cancer, the Gunthers combed each day's news-papers and pursued every possibility, from conventional surgery to dietary regimens of dubious value.[1]

It is indeed possible that a search of such intensity occasionally brings the patient additional years of life. But for most people who develop cancer, treatment by competent professionals applying standard techniques offers the best chance for survival. This will be as true in the twenty-first century as it was at the time this book was written. Far into the future, the ability to obtain well-planned, skillfully applied, but nevertheless standard care will make the basic difference in who survives.

To help demonstrate this crucial point, this chapter provides a glimpse at the practice and development of cancer treatment methods.

This prescription for survival does not sound heroic. The term *standard techniques* refers to conventional treatment modalities utilized by cancer specialists throughout the United States. For the majority of patients with most forms of cancer, such treatment will constitute appropriate care. More novel and intensive intervention than the normal standard of care provides little material benefit to most. Such intervention includes both experimental treatment that may take place at major research facilities and "alternative" forms of therapy provided by unorthodox practitioners. Practitioners in these sectors of the health care industry may possess extraordinary skills in some areas important to cancer patients. The research setting may provide better technical services in some areas. The unorthodox practitioner may offer great emotional support. But neither experimental nor unorthodox treatment seems likely to extend the lives of most patients to a significant degree.

This is not to say that standard therapy for cancer is simple or straightforward. As the previous chapter indicates, cancer is a highly complex category of diseases with important variations even in major anatomical sites. The nature of appropriate treatment may vary from case to case more widely than in any other illness. While some routine principles apply to every patient, it seems likely that many lives have been saved or lost as a result of the quality of decisions in individual cases. This principle applies to the activities of health professionals in the accuracy of diagnostic judgment, acuity and dexterity in treatment, care in monitoring, and encouragement of the patient. It applies to efficiency in communication and scheduling of procedures in the medical practice or hospital. The patient cannot assume without question that his or her family physician or community hospital can indeed provide the most appropriate care. But neither can the patient assume that a practitioner or facility offering unusually intensive treatment or a unique approach to care will achieve better results.

This chapter reviews issues in cancer treatment likely to be most important to the informed patient. It provides basic information about conventional forms of care—those of most practical significance for the average cancer patient—and the logic that physicians use in applying related techniques. It discusses some of the major currents in cancer research and assesses the benefits an average patient may gain by becoming an experimental subject. It takes an objective look at some of the principal forms of unorthodox treatment to which patients turned in the late twentieth century. It inquires about the potential contributions that research may ultimately make to curing cancer.

This review serves as a foundation for the major message of this book: For most individuals with cancer, survival depends primarily on gaining access to good, conventional treatment—a process dependent on both personal initiative and resources for health care. Neither the possibility of major scientific "breakthroughs" nor the availability of unorthodox treatment offers significant near-term benefits to many cancer patients. The process of conventional care, however, is hardly routine or trivial, as a brief exploration of its practice demonstrates. Ensuring that this practice takes place in a reliable manner and that most patients enjoy timely access to it may require basic rethinking of the arrangements under which Americans received and paid for their health care in the late twentieth century.

The Practice of Conventional Care

Whether treated in community hospitals or world-famous medical centers, most cancer patients receive well-tested treatments developed through years of research and honed in clinical experience. Almost always, these will consist of surgery, radiation therapy, chemotherapy, or some combination of these interventions. Appropriate care requires tailoring the application of individual or combination therapies to the specifics of each case. In applying these treatment modalities, physicians must resolve questions peculiar to each. Some dilemmas, moreover, apply to all cancer treatments.

CONVENTIONAL TREATMENT MODALITIES

Readers unfamiliar with cancer treatment will benefit from a brief review of the major modalities in use around 1990. Even a minimum amount of information about the approaches and procedures used to treat cancer makes discussion of the associated choices and dilemmas much more meaningful. This review is intended to provide sufficient background for nonspecialists to understand how an individual's decisions and the conditions under which he or she receives care may affect survival. It constitutes only a fleeting look at surgery, radiation therapy, and chemotherapy. Detailed technical information on cancer treatment and on therapeutic options for specific malignancies is beyond the scope of this book. Likewise, this discussion omits several important though relatively unusual approaches to treatment. Later discussion will address some of these modalities. Those seeking more detailed or comprehensive information may consult one of the textbooks available on cancer treatment;[2] scientific and medical journals that include articles on cancer research and therapy are published worldwide, and doubtless number in the hundreds.

Surgery. Surgery is the most basic, oldest, and still most often used method in the treatment of cancer. The most frankly invasive of therapies, surgery imparts an aura of heroism to both doctor and patient. The years between 1880 and 1950 saw a steady increase in reliability and popularity of surgical treatment for cancer as well as many other conditions. Basic progress in biology and medicine stood behind these advances. During this era, aseptic methods became available to reduce the extreme hazard of infection. Anesthesia became less risky. Surgeons learned to manage shock, blood loss, and respiratory problems during and after operations. All these advances allowed surgeons to perform longer operations and carry out more complex procedures.

Historically, the rationale behind cancer surgery appears simple: remove the malignant growth as completely and rapidly as possible to relieve interference with normal function and forestall the possibility of metastatic spread. This classical approach was embodied in the surgical procedure for breast cancer developed by William Halsted, a great pioneer of the late nineteenth century. The Halsted procedure consisted of radical mastectomy, including removal of the breast, underlying muscle, and nearby lymph nodes. Halsted believed that the principal danger of cancer dissemination occurred by direct movement of malignant disease from the original lesion to surrounding tissues and anatomical structures.[3] Today's specialists know that tissues far removed from the original lesion may be at greater risk and that those relatively nearby may remain unaffected. However, surgeons followed the basic outlines of Halsted's radical mastectomy procedure well into the 1950s.

In actual practice, cancer surgery is by no means simple. Every patient who undergoes extensive surgery risks death from general anesthesia. Surgeons carry out procedures that vary widely among patients, and often make complicated treatment decisions during the operation itself. Different surgical procedures will be performed depending on the location of the tumor and the apparent dissemination of the disease.

Dissemination of disease, furthermore, is a matter not only of extent and distance from the original lesion but also of pattern of spread. In some diseases, surgical procedures may themselves cause cancer cells to spread; surgeons must use special procedures to guard against this possibility. Surgeons do not always agree about which procedures are most effective given the specifics of a malignancy. As one authority has commented, the selection of an actual procedure "usually rests upon 'surgical judgement,' and great variation or even arbitrary selection of a surgical approach occurs."[4]

Radiation. Use of radiation to treat cancer dates from the late nineteenth century, following soon after the discovery of X rays in 1895 and of natural radiation in 1896. Radiation consists of high-energy waves or particles produced by electromagnetic devices (e.g., high-voltage vacuum tubes) or radioactive elements and their compounds. Very high-energy radiation has the capacity to produce ionization, knocking electrons out of their atomic orbits in matter that it strikes. Ionizing radiation includes waves, such as X rays and gamma rays, and particles, such as neutrons and protons. Only ionizing radiation is used in cancer therapy and, as late as the 1980s, only waves. In the late twentieth century, devices using conventional X-ray tubes and cobalt-60 sources of radiation were largely replaced by much higher-energy equipment, such as linear accelerators. Higher-energy sources produce more penetrating, sharply focused radiation beams, delivering more destructive power to diseased areas while sparing healthy tissue from exposure.

When absorbed by living tissue, radiation causes death or damage to the cells. Much of a cell is composed of water, from which radiation produces a variety of compounds and ionized particles. While short-lived, these particles rapidly combine with cell proteins, interfering with their normal function in the cell. Ionizing radiation produces compounds that break apart DNA, vital for cell reproduction. Radiation destroys cancer tissue by killing individual cells or limiting their ability to reproduce. Tumors do not seem to be able to maintain themselves if a significant proportion of their cells lose the ability to replicate.

Doctors have several options for delivering radiation to a tumor. Those most often used are external beams generated by electromagnetic devices or implants containing radioactive substances placed inside the body. External beam therapy can deliver radiation through the skin and other tissues, concentrating greatest energy on the specific internal location targeted for therapy. Focusing beams from several angles results in concentration at the desired spot while sparing healthy tissue.

Interstitial radiation therapy involves implantation of a radioactive source within the body in close proximity to the diseased tissue. In treating prostate cancer, for example, physicians may implant radioactive gold or iodine in the form of seeds or needlelike stilettes in the tissue bed from which a tumor has been removed. These implants deliver radioactivity to the exact area desired and continue doing so for months without interruption.[5] Physicians may implant grains of radioactive material near tumors in deep-lying organs such as the liver, threading catheters bearing these materials through large veins to reach their targets.

While radiation may play the primary role in treatment of some cancers, it is often used as a follow-up procedure for surgery. Physicians may perform radiation therapy to treat malignant tissue that surgeons are not able to remove. In addition, radiation may be used as "adjuvant" therapy; that is, treatment for disease that is not apparent but is suspected of existing or thought likely to develop at a later time. Patients receiving surgery for mouth cancers, for example, may later receive radiation therapy to nearby lymph nodes, even though they show no signs of metastases. Patients with small cell lung cancer may receive prophylactic radiation to the skull. The brain is a frequent target of metastases in this form of cancer, and resulting brain dysfunctions often prove the immediate cause of death.

Radiation therapy does not have the same heroic panache as surgery. External beam therapy is almost always performed on an outpatient basis; the patient receives this therapy in a specially designed room, awake, and often standing up. He or she usually sees, hears, and smells nothing extraordinary during the procedure, which is conducted as a series of treatments repeated over several weeks. Radioactive implants may be placed after the removal of a tumor in surgery but may also be deposited in nonsurgical procedures.

While less apparently intrusive than surgery, radiation has a powerful impact on the body. As in surgery, medical judgment is required to determine when and what kind of radiation may be beneficial. Radiation causes a variety of side effects, including loss of appetite, nausea, and damage to the linings of the esophagus and intestines. The mechanisms by which radiation therapy damages cells, moreover, can themselves give rise to cancer; patients undergoing radiation therapy have been known to develop additional tumors as a result of their treatment. Physicians can reduce the immediate side effects of radiation therapy by scheduling intervals for recovery between radiation dosages.

Chemotherapy. The newest of the major cancer treatment modalities, chemotherapy involves treatment with drugs that destroy cancer cells. This form of treatment has been said to owe its origins to the explosion of an Allied ship carrying mustard gas during World War II. According to autopsies of soldiers on the ship, exposure to the gas had inhibited production of white blood cells. This finding led to speculation that the gas might prove useful in treating leukemia and other blood and lymph cancers characterized by a proliferation of abnormal white cells.[6] Others trace the beginnings of chemotherapy to the early 1940s, when C. Huggins and C. V. Hodges at the University of Chicago discovered that administration of female hormones to men with prostate cancer inhibited tumor growth.

Throughout the middle and late twentieth century, chemotherapy maintained a special appeal for American science. A form of drug treatment, chemotherapy recalled the successes that had revolutionized medicine between the late nineteenth century and World War II, when penicillin, sulfa drugs, and antibiotics brought many infectious diseases under control.

Patients receive chemotherapy in a manner similar to that employed in other drug regimens—usually via infusion or injection or, less frequently, oral medication. They often receive the medication via intravenous line in a hospital or a physician's office. The timing of a course of chemotherapy is similar to that of radiation therapy, usually lasting several weeks or months with periodic breaks. The administration of many chemotherapeutic agents requires the use of precision pumping devices to ensure the infusion of drugs at the prescribed rate.

Chemotherapy serves as the primary treatment for several forms of cancer, particularly those in which surgery is inappropriate. These include cancers that do not form "solid" tumors (for instance, leukemia) and cancers that are widely disseminated throughout the body (for instance, lymphoma). Chemotherapy is the only feasible treatment for cancers that are widely disseminated throughout the body. Use of chemotherapy has raised the life expectancies of persons with small cell lung cancer, a highly aggressive malignancy seldom found without having metastasized.[7] Adjuvant chemotherapy has proven especially beneficial in some malignancies, particularly cancer of the breast. However, scientists have been much less successful in developing chemotherapeutic agents for several frequently occurring cancers, including colon, prostate, pancreatic, cervical, bladder, and lung cancer other than small cell.[8]

All chemotherapeutic agents either kill cancer cells, inhibit their development, or prevent them from reproducing. Most agents produce these effects by preventing cancer cells from making DNA, or by preventing this substance from playing its required role in the cell. The agents may block access to nutrients needed to make DNA, damage the DNA's chemical structure, or prevent its action on other chemicals within the cell. Some forms of chemotherapy have much in common with radiation therapy. Radiation causes "alkylating agents" to form within the cell and lock onto DNA strands, thus preventing their normal operation. Alkylating agents are one of the most important families of drugs used in chemotherapy.

While it does not involve the drama of the operating room or the space-age machinery of the radiology unit, chemotherapy is a very complex and hazardous endeavor, requiring a high level of expertise and attention to detail from the physician. It is hazardous because all chemotherapeutic agents—other than hormones, which in any case are sometimes considered a different form of therapy—are cytotoxic, or poisonous. They may attack tumors, but they also devastate normal tissues. The DNA of normal and cancer cells differs in only the most minute detail. Chemicals that interfere with vital functions in cancer cells interfere with these same functions in normal cells. Chemotherapeutic drugs may exercise "selective toxicity" only because they affect cells at a specific point in their life cycle. Thus, a drug may damage a tumor more extensively than a normal organ because a greater proportion of cancer cells, which reproduce rapidly, pass this point in the life cycle. Normal cells, however, are also vulnerable, and many are injured or die. The cells that normally reproduce rapidly in the body—including bone marrow, linings of the intestines, and hair follicles—bear the brunt of this damage, giving rise to side effects such as anemia, diarrhea, and hair loss.

Another problem with chemotherapy is that malignant cell masses tend to develop resistance to chemotherapeutic drugs. Like bacteria exposed to antibiotics, malignant tissues harbor some cells that have natural resistance to many of these agents. Although the chemotherapeutic agents initially affect most cells, those that are immune survive, eventually giving rise to a drug-resistant tumor. This process is accelerated by the tendency of cancer cells to mutate with ever greater frequency as the tumor develops, the entire cell mass "mutating toward" immunity. For many cancers, researchers have formulated chemotherapeutic regimens combining several different drugs, some given simultaneously, others in sequence. This strategy helps combat cancer cell immunity and may provide the patient with periodic respite from the most toxic agents.

Chemotherapy requires the physician to become a strategist, continuously assessing the response of an individual disease to specific agents and regimens, and monitoring the patient's tolerance of the drugs. The side effects of this form of cancer treatment go well beyond nausea and hair loss and may become life-threatening in themselves. The patient may become exhausted because loss of appetite has led to malnutrition; bone marrow poisoning may undermine resistance to infectious disease; lung damage, kidney dysfunction, and hemorrhage may occur. The physician often must reformulate the combination of drugs used and recalibrate their dosage. As in so much of medicine, effective treatment becomes as much art as science.

Most cancer patients at the end of the twentieth century received surgery, radiation, chemotherapy, or some combination of these interventions. Many received other treatments as well. Immunotherapy, an intervention designed to strengthen the body's natural capabilities for fighting cancer, created significant excitement as an experimental field. Others, such as treatment with vitamins and Laetrile, fell under headings such as "alternative" or "unorthodox." Glamorous areas such as these grabbed headlines. But less newsworthy concerns faced thousands of cancer patients in these years; practical decisions related to accepted forms of treatment determine ultimate survival. Individual choices among accepted therapies represent key crossroads for most patients, profoundly affecting both life expectancy and quality.

CONSERVATIVE VERSUS AGGRESSIVE INTERVENTION: A KEY TREATMENT DECISION

For most people who develop cancer, survival depends on appropriate use of conventional surgery, radiation therapy, and chemotherapy. Cancer, of course, represents hundreds if not thousands of different disease syndromes. The delineation of appropriate care for even a few of these syndromes would be complex and highly technical. But the importance of appropriate care and the challenges of determining an appropriate course of treatment are illustrated by one of many dilemmas that regularly face physicians and patients: conservative versus aggressive intervention. In this context, *conservative* refers to the use of limited procedures focused primarily on visible disease and having minimum impact on the patient's overall condition. *Aggressive* indicates the use of extensive interventions, necessarily affecting the patient's overall functioning in a material way.

Physicians and patients alike feel pressure to choose aggressive treatment. A nation of activists, Americans typically want their physicians to bring the full force of the medical arsenal to bear, even where the impacts of treatment are often severe and the benefits uncertain. A medically correct decision may still result in ill feelings. When a patient dies, having refused an available though dubious treatment, loved ones may comment, "The doctor let him die." Recalling after another death the deterioration of a patient under intensive, desperate therapy, survivors may remark, "The doctor killed him."

The basic biology of cancer makes dilemmas such as this unavoidable. Scientists of the early twentieth century developed "magic bullets" to fight infectious disease. Like antibiotics on bacteria or weakened polio viruses on the immune system, these agents usually destroyed disease-causing organisms or enabled the body to build up defenses against future exposures without major effects on normal tissues or processes. The cancer specialists of the twentieth century possessed no magic bullets to kill cancer cells while leaving normal ones intact. Despite their inability to perform normal functions and their aberrant morphology, cancer cells share almost every basic biological characteristic of normal cells. No intervention effective at the cellular level has a true specific toxicity to cancer, damaging malignant cells yet sparing normal ones. As the surgeon's knife excises not only malignant but normal tissue, so do radiation and chemotherapy necessarily destroy normal cells.

In balancing destruction of malignant tissue against injury to the patient, clinicians face case-by-case choices between conservative and aggressive treatment. Conservative treatment tends to depend on a single modality (surgery *or* radiation) and a limited application of the technique. This procedure leaves normal structures and tissues relatively unharmed but may expose the patient to risk of recurrent disease. Aggressive treatment often involves a multimodal approach, combining, for example, surgery with radiation. An aggressive surgical procedure removes more tissue; an aggressive chemotherapy program administers drugs in higher dosages or of greater toxicity. Although aggressive treatment aims at reducing the reappearance of disease at a later time, its side effects may endanger the patient and leave him or her with dysfunction or disfigurement even if it brings about permanent cure.

In deciding whether to undertake aggressive or conservative treatment, patients and physicians often must balance chances for cure against undesired side effects. In other instances, aggressive treatment is wholly inappropriate because it is ineffective in enhancing chances for survival.

Exemplifying aggressive surgery, Halsted's radical mastectomy raises additional treatment issues. As described above, this nineteenth-century innovation for breast cancer removed not only the tumor but also underlying muscle tissue and nearby lymph nodes. Practiced for even limited disease well into the twentieth century, the radical mastectomy terrified generations of women, who perceived loss of a breast as profound disfigurement. In the 1960s and 1970s, an increasing number of surgeons began performing more limited procedures. New operations spared the muscle underlying the breast and thus a significant portion of the breast itself. Long-term studies indicated that women with early breast cancer who underwent the more limited procedure had chances for survival comparable to those with radical mastectomies.[9] Women diagnosed with breast cancer at any stage may now discuss several options with their physicians, balancing cosmetic considerations against what often amount to very small survival advantages with aggressive surgery.

A review of recent research in prostate cancer treatment reveals a similar set of trade-offs between conservative and aggressive treatment. Physicians and patients face vexing choices in selecting among options for therapy. Though often a slow-moving malignancy, prostate cancer is a truly life-threatening disease, especially when it strikes younger men.[10] Aggressive treatment may increase survival chances for some, although at potentially high cost in function and self-image. For other patients, aggressive treatment may only hasten death.

Perhaps no area of cancer treatment in the late twentieth century has involved more controversy among physicians than radical surgery for prostate cancer. A curative procedure, radical prostatectomy removes the entire prostate gland, with the objective of excising the entire lesion before metastasis begins. This aggressive surgical procedure may include placement of radioactive implants in the tumor bed to fight malignant cells that may remain. Some physicians, however, believe that the spread of prostate cancer, though slow, is inexorable. According to this interpretation, radical surgery is seldom if ever curative, since the disease has already spread by the time it is discovered. Physicians holding this view believe that the benefits of radical surgery do not justify their costs to the patient in side effects and risks. Some may operate if the tumor is extremely small and its cells are of undifferentiated histology, known to disseminate aggressively. Others may attempt cure by treating the tumor with external beam radiation while it is still localized. Still others prefer to watch and wait, perhaps ordering external beam radiation therapy if and when the tumor shows actual signs of spreading.

Several important studies of early prostate cancer published in the 1980s supported the strategy of aggressive surgery. Based on review of medical records, one study found that men who received the radical surgery had an almost 25 percent greater chance of surviving for fifteen years than those who received radiation therapy.[11] This study, however, was unable to assign patients randomly to each treatment setting, a practice widely regarded as necessary for valid results. A study that did randomly assign men with early prostate cancer to radical surgery versus radiation found that those who received radiation were more likely to develop cancer outside the prostate itself. But this study did not find differences in actual survival.[12]

While a consensus in favor of radical surgery may have been developing in the 1980s, its benefits were still equivocal. The procedure involves significant side effects. Because radical surgery removes the nerves and blood vessels required for erection, many men lost sexual function. Many also experienced at least partial loss of bladder control.

A potentially important series of studies of prostatic cancer suggests an additional need for judgment in applying "standard" treatments. The transurethral resection of the prostate, or TURP, is used widely to relieve urinary retention. TURP involves removing only enough of the prostate gland (which surrounds the urethra) to permit the free flow of urine. However, evidence has surfaced that in localized (though clinically evident) prostate cancer, TURP may actually spread cancer cells and result in early mortality.[13] This hazard is apparently not present in later-stage disease, where urinary retention may also develop. If these reports are correct, a seemingly limited procedure would turn into a very dangerous one unless accurate determination of disease stage was made before the surgery.

Administration of female hormones, another important treatment for prostate cancer, involves other trade-offs. As the landmark research by Huggins and Hodges in the early 1940s indicated, male sex hormones stimulate the growth of malignant prostate tumors. As a result of these findings, physicians developed therapies designed to reduce the concentration of male hormones in the bloodstreams of patients with advanced prostate cancer. Administration of female hormone may accomplish this effect, causing the testes to stop secreting male hormone.

Ironically, however, such aggressive drug therapy may not prolong life. A major Veterans Administration study suggested that control of prostate cancer achieved through high doses of female hormone may be neutralized by an increased risk of heart attacks.[14] A surgical alternative to prescription of female hormone is castration (orchiectomy). While this procedure may reduce risk from heart attacks, many men find it difficult to accept.

Lung cancer, the most frequently diagnosed and most widely lethal malignancy in the United States, also illustrates dilemmas in conservative versus aggressive treatment. Several convincing studies indicate that aggressive treatment indeed prolongs life. This finding is well documented in early-stage, non–small cell lung cancer, where patients apparently obtain cures through surgery. According to one study, 53 percent of patients with Stage I and 29 percent of patients with Stage II disease remained alive five years after surgery.[15] Small cell lung cancer, the most rapidly metastatic form of the disease, responds to chemotherapy. A study of an especially aggressive regimen reported that up to 15 percent of patients who received a combination of several powerful chemotherapeutic agents plus radiation survived two years or longer. For those receiving only radiation or single-agent chemotherapy, two-year survival was 2 percent or less.[16]

These impressive survival reports, however, must be balanced against the risks of treatment. In surgery for non–small cell lung cancer, the frequency of postoperative surgical death—that is, death within thirty days of surgery, probably due to the impact of surgery itself—parallels the aggressiveness of the procedure. A large-scale study in the early 1980s indicated that 6.2 percent of lung cancer patients died during or soon after surgery to remove an entire lung; the figure was 2.9 percent for removal of a lobe of the affected lung, a less aggressive procedure.[17] The achievements of aggressive care for small cell lung cancer must be balanced against the realization that the addition of radiation to chemotherapy does not apparently extend survival; a nearly equal proportion (about 10 percent) of those treated only with chemotherapy and chemotherapy plus radiation remained alive and disease-free after two years.[18]

Studies of treatment in other cancers raise further warnings about the benefits of aggressive care. Women with Stage I adenocarcinoma of the cervix were reported to have had a 52 percent five-year survival rate if they received only radiation therapy, and an 83 percent five-year survival rate if they received radiation plus radical hysterectomy. But some investigators reported that patients whose care included surgery also experienced complications much more frequently.[19] Aggressive treatment for pancreatic cancer raises the issue of conservative versus aggressive treatment in a particularly stark fashion. A commentator questioned the use of Whipple resection, a surgical procedure for pancreatic cancer that involves the removal of several internal organs, noting that of 15,000 patients reported to have undergone such surgery, only 65 survived five years.[20]

This brief review of standard cancer treatments has two basic messages. First, it appears that no treatment for cancer is, in fact, entirely standard. The physician's judgment and the patient's choice play important parts in determining survival. Second, more intensive use of the conventional treatment modalities is not necessarily beneficial. Even given the same extent of disease, the patient who receives the more extensive operation or the more potent chemotherapy does not necessarily live longer.

Experimental Therapy

For many cancer patients, the search for a cure ends with entry into an experiment. Patients often receive conventional treatment through several episodes of their illness, surviving successive remissions and recurrences. Generally, experimental treatment becomes appropriate when the cancer no longer responds to any of these interventions or the patient can no longer tolerate standard modalities. Medical and scientific ethics forbid treating patients with experimental methods before this time. Thus, experimental treatment may represent the patient's last hope. Many patients who have exhausted all conventional treatment hunt frantically for doctors investigating new therapies and ask to be considered as experimental subjects. Some experience keen disappointment as their conditions or personal characteristics prove incompatible with the experimental design, and they are rejected.

But for most individual patients, experimental treatment in fact offers few material benefits. To enthusiastic believers in science, especially those faced with terminal illness, the word *experiment* connotes innovation, progress, the betterment of life. To physicians and scientists engaged in trials of unproven therapies, such interventions seem to be viewed much more skeptically. A trial of interleukin-2 (IL-2), a preparation formulated to boost the immune system's ability to destroy cancer cells, provides illustrations of these differing perspectives. According to a cancer patient in the experiment who had previously failed to respond to chemotherapy,

> I am making a firm prediction that interleukin-2 will bring me out of it.
>
> Compared to chemotherapy, this is a piece of cake. All I have to do to get well is face a half hour of discomfort, of needle-jabbing.
>
> I'm tickled pink to be part of a study because so much of your macho dignity is taken away [in chemotherapy]. Now the dignity is being returned. And, if through my getting well, I can be of service—Lord, I'm just so appreciative.

But according to the doctor conducting the trial, "Honestly, my expectations are limited."[21]

Basic science and experimental treatment play an important part in cancer therapy today and have profound implications for the future. But more immediate questions require attention as well. How does, and to what extent will, cancer research improve cancer treatment? What benefits can *today's* cancer patients draw from these experiments?

CURRENT SCIENTIFIC INVESTIGATIONS

Every day, thousands of Americans with advanced cancer help test new therapies. Many of the techniques under study are refinements and extensions of established treatments. In the late twentieth century, for example, significant work continued on new kinds of radiation therapy, including experimentation with radioactive implants for fighting tumors in the brain, breast, and kidney.

The largest number of experiments during this era probably involved chemotherapy. By the 1970s, chemotherapy had become a very effective treatment for leukemia and other diseases of the blood and lymph systems and had proven useful for some solid tumors as well.[22] Scientists were eager to extend this technology to additional forms of cancer, and continuously tested new drugs, new combinations of old drugs, and new methods of injecting or infusing already familiar medications. Much research on chemotherapy involved the testing of drug analogs, new compounds that differed from the old ones only by the presence, absence, or placement of a few atoms or groups of atoms in a large molecular structure. The first chemotherapeutic agents found to be effective against lymphoma required the testing of 1,500 analogs of nitrogen mustard and other alkylating agents.

Immunotherapy seemed to be creating the most excitement among scientists as a fundamentally new form of cancer treatment. For decades, scientists had wondered why the body's natural immune system did not destroy cancer cells as it did bacteria and other foreign bodies. They theorized that strengthening the natural immune system would allow the body to fight off cancer. In the early 1900s, scientists injected cancer patients with specially cultured strains of bacteria (including one form of tuberculosis) and toxins prepared from bacterial cultures in attempts to stimulate the immune system to the point where it would become effective against cancer cells.

With the advent of genetic engineering in the 1970s, scientists began developing several entirely new approaches to immunotherapy. A fascinating example is adoptive immunotherapy. Through genetic engineering, scientists manufactured a class of agents called *biological response modifiers*.[23] When certain white blood cells were exposed to these substances, they became very aggressive. In the 1980s, scientists began experimenting with biological response modifiers called lymphokines, such as IL-2. Exposure of white blood cells to lymphokines created lymphokine-activated killer (LAK) cells capable of fighting tumors. LAK cells could be created from the patient's own white blood cells in two ways. Biological response modifiers could be injected into the patient to stimulate the development of the cells within his or her body. Alternatively, cells could be removed from the body, exposed to a substance such as IL-2, and returned to the body after activation. Experiments were conducted to determine the effectiveness of many possible treatment approaches.

THE PROCESS OF RESEARCH

Whether it involves biological response modifiers, chemotherapy, or any other conventional or unconventional form of treatment, cancer research is a complex, time-consuming, and expensive process. A single research effort may require the participation of hundreds of patients, who must be selected carefully, treated in a uniform manner, and monitored closely. Some of this research is conducted by the government at the National Institutes of Health, but much more often it takes place at medical research centers affiliated with universities. More and more often, several such research centers combine to carry out an experiment. This cooperation is necessary, in part, because a single center, even if very large, may not see enough patients with the desired characteristics to conduct a successful experiment. Reports by coalitions of scientists—for example, ECOG (Eastern Cooperative Oncology Group), SWOG (Southwest Oncology Group), and the Lung Cancer Study Group—appear with ever greater frequency in the medical journals. In the 1980s, the federal government initiated the Community Clinical Oncology Program (CCOP) with the objective of bringing physicians outside academic medical centers into the research process. This program aimed at increasing the pool of experimental subjects, making new treatment options available to more patients, and speeding the flow of information from the research center to the practitioner community.[24]

The first steps in developing a new treatment occur in the laboratory, years before patients become involved. Chemotherapy provides a good example of the early stages of cancer research. Drawing on their general knowledge of the biological activity of various chemicals, clinical experience, and educated guesswork, scientists identify compounds they believe may be active against cancer. They then expose mice that harbor cancer cells to these substances and study the tumor response. These mice are especially bred to have extremely weak immune systems, so that the tumor response, if any, may be attributed only to the experimental substance. The cancer cells implanted in the mice are of a type that mimics the characteristics of human malignancies. If the tumors shrink or disappear, and the substance does not prove too toxic, the scientists may move on to human experimentation.

Government agencies and research institutions have developed strict rules and traditions for conducting cancer research on human beings. Such regulation befits a field of key scientific interest regularly confronting life-and-death situations. Conventions for the conduct and supervision of research involving patients represent attempts to ensure that scientists take adequate steps to produce valid findings and protect patients from harm.

Human experimentation, also known as clinical trials, usually takes place in three stages. In Phase I, scientists administer the experimental substance to a group of patients to determine the maximum dosage that can be administered safely. Patients are monitored carefully for side effects.

In Phase II, the research question shifts from safety to effectiveness. The researchers administer the maximum safely tolerated dose to a group of cancer patients for whom no other therapy has been effective. Individuals with several different cancers may be involved. They are followed to determine whether their tumors disappear, shrink, or otherwise respond to the therapy. Scientists continue to monitor patients for side effects during the Phase II trial.

Phase III most strongly resembles a classical scientific experiment. In this phase, cancer patients are randomly assigned to several alternative treatments, known as "arms" of the study. All of these treatments must be presumed to be of equal efficacy for the individual patient's disease. Various arms of the study may consist of a standard treatment or other experimental therapies. When no other standard or experimental treatment exists, scientists may give some of the patients a placebo, a substance known not to affect the tumor. Patients are carefully observed to determine whether the new treatment offers any advantage over treatments already in use. If the treatment is found to have an overall therapeutic advantage—such as tumor remission, enhanced survival, or decreased toxicity in comparison with alternatives—it is licensed for marketing and may be used freely by practitioners in the community.

There is no guarantee, of course, that scientists will move smoothly from phase to phase in the experimental process. The federal Food and Drug Administration must grant permission to use any drug, device, or biological product for a Phase I trial. Universities, hospitals, and other research facilities have institutional review boards to examine experimental plans and procedures, and human subjects committees to ensure that experimental patients are properly informed of the risks and benefits of the proposed investigational treatments. The National Institutes of Health, which funds most biomedical research in the United States, exercises oversight when it reviews requests for research grants and requires organizations that receive such grants to hold internal reviews. Review of experimental findings takes place at every phase, and the process stops at whatever point the experimental treatment is found to be too toxic for human consumption or fails to provide evidence of advantages over established techniques.

DOES THE EXPERIMENTAL TREATMENT BENEFIT THE PATIENT?

Most patients know little if anything about the scientific planning of the experiments in which they are involved—they simply desire a cure. For many, participation does not come cheap. The medical center at which experimental treatment takes place may be far from home, reducing contact with loved ones in the last days and weeks of life.

The treatment may involve significant discomfort. Monitoring may require frequent drawing of blood and other tests. Ordinarily, the patient continues to pay for much if not all of his or her health care.

How much extension of life do those who receive experimental treatment actually obtain? Any survival advantage seems to be, on average, very small. Many new interventions prove no more effective than conventional treatments. Those that turn out to be superior seldom result in the hoped-for cures. Average life extension in those experiments that are successful is usually measured in weeks or months rather than years.

Several clinical trials in prostate and lung cancer illustrate the elusiveness of life extension through experimental treatment. Because the standard diethylstilbestrol (DES) treatment of advanced prostate cancer exposes the patient to risk of heart attack, scientists have sought alternative forms of chemotherapy. In one randomized study, patients with advanced prostate cancer whose diseases were not controlled by surgery, estrogens, or orchiectomy (castration) were placed on alternative chemotherapy regimens. Neither group evidenced any particular extension of life.[25] Another study compared survival among patients with advanced prostate cancer randomly assigned to treatment with DES and two alternative hormones. Survival was equal among those receiving DES and one of the two alternative treatments; survival was *lower* among patients receiving the second alternative.[26]

Scientists may have carried out more clinical trials for lung cancer than for any other malignancy. Development of effective forms of chemotherapy for small cell lung cancer has encouraged the search for agents effective against the more common non–small cell varieties. In the late twentieth century, patients with this disease obtained no survival advantages by joining clinical trials. Phase III trials conducted in the 1970s and 1980s found some responses to new therapies—shrinkage of tumors, for example—but no improvements in survival.[27] Side effects from some of these regimens proved fatal, various drugs causing patients to die from hemorrhage, kidney failure, infections, and general exhaustion. One researcher concluded, "Currently, the choice of therapy for metastatic [non–small cell] lung cancer rests more on an analysis of toxicity rather than on response and survival."[28]

Experimentation on patients with small cell lung cancer has been more successful. Between 1973 and 1978, treatment with aggressive chemotherapy and radiation improved the survival chances of people with this disease. One of the most important advances in treatment of small cell lung cancer was replacement of single-agent chemotherapy with regimens utilizing combinations of drugs. This development in the standard of care added an average of five months to the lives of small cell lung cancer patients.[29] Participants in trials that led to this development added, on the average, a fraction of this number of months to their lives. It is unlikely that anyone with small cell lung cancer added to his or her survival by participating in a chemotherapy trial after 1978, since progress in this area seemed to have reached a plateau. In one radiation therapy trial, patients with small cell lung cancer did experience increased survival, but only by an average of about one month in the most successful arm of the experiment.[30]

Results of major clinical trials of adoptive immunotherapy began to appear in the medical journals in the late 1980s. These studies treated patients with IL-2 plus LAK cells or with high doses of IL-2 alone. They included only patients who had failed to respond to standard treatment or for whom no standard treatment was available. Although 25 percent responded to treatment, their tumors shrinking or disappearing, no information on survival was yet available.[31] As late as 1990, a scientific advisory panel of the Food and Drug Administration refused to recommend licensing of IL-2 as a standard drug.[32] The Cetus Corporation, the drug's manufacturer, claimed that IL-2 was effective against kidney cancer, for which there was no alternative treatment. Alarmed at its toxicity, however, several panel members requested that Cetus demonstrate *which* kidney cancer patients would actually benefit. According to several panel members, the drug was so toxic that only patients with disease characteristics ideal for IL-2 would obtain a net benefit from its use.

A cancer patient hoping that an experimental treatment will produce a cure can learn much from this brief overview. Very few people are "cured" in the traditional sense by experimental interventions. People who have exhausted all conventional therapies seldom extend their lives to a significant degree through these experiments. Particularly promising experimental interventions may add months to the lives of some patients, though often at significant cost in money and discomfort. Rarely, a patient on a clinical trial will live for many years beyond expectations, perhaps because the treatment given *just happens* to prove ideal for his or her individual tumor, through inexplicable good luck.

Generally, experimental treatment is not the key to survival for individual cancer patients. The best reason to participate in a trial may be to perform public service. Although the individual may gain little additional life from experimental treatment, his or her participation may help extend the lives of others. Most effective cancer treatments have come about through evolution rather than breakthroughs. Early use of nitrogen mustard brought limited life extension to a few lymphoma patients; in later trials, new drugs added to the regimen increased the length of survival and raised the percentage of patients favorably affected. Similar step-by-step processes yielded standard therapies for cancers of the breast, ovaries, and testes, as well as small cell lung cancer. Small or negligible gains for individuals, then, may add up to significant therapeutic improvement over the long run. But patients should never expect to enter an experiment just in time for the "breakthrough," which, if the history and development of cancer treatment accurately portend, will never come.

Alternative Cures

People with serious illnesses have always sought cures for their conditions outside mainstream medicine. Characterizing the nineteenth century as the "golden age of quackery," Barrie Cassileth describes some of the era's popular cancer nostrums and their present-day successors:

Early in the 1900s, cancer-targeted quasi-medicines in pill or liquid form appeared, such as Radol, Chamlee's Cancer-Specific Purifies-the-Blood Cure, and a host of others. During the then-new electronic age of radio, telegraph, telephone, and other miracles produced by energy, the 1920s saw "energy" cancer cures such as "cosmic energy treatment" and "light therapy." Koch's glyoxilide (distilled water) cure of the 1940s was followed by the Hoxsey Treatment in extract and pill form in the 1950s, by injectable Krebiozen during the 1960s, and by Laetrile in the 1970s. Each, in its own time, created a furor and a degree of media exposure at least equal to that aroused recently by Laetrile.[33]

According to Cassileth, the most popular alternative treatments in the late twentieth century included "metabolic" and diet therapies. These treatments are alleged to cure cancer by removing toxins from the body and providing cells with the nutrients they need to function and maintain health. The belief that massive doses of vitamin C can cure cancer also attained a large following at this time.

The superstitious and ignorant have always availed themselves of "quack" cures; the unscrupulous have always made these cures available for profit. But many alternative therapies in the late twentieth century attracted a following among the educated; several, moreover, were developed and popularized by leading scientists.

Krebiozen attracted a large following in the 1950s and early 1960s. Introduced in the United States by Dr. Steven Durovic, a Yugoslav refugee, Krebiozen proved on analysis to be a highly diluted preparation of horse meat in mineral oil. The American Medical Association characterized Krebiozen as "one of the greatest frauds of the 20th century." Yet one of the drug's leading public supporters was Dr. Andrew Ivy, a highly respected scientist and professor at the University of Illinois. Ivy had served as chairman of a key policy-making body at the National Cancer Institute, a unit of the National Institutes of Health, which makes large-scale funding available to cancer scientists and thus predominates in setting the direction of cancer research and treatment nationwide. Senator Paul Douglas of Illinois sponsored legislation to allow Dr. Durovic to remain in the United States and urged the government to give Krebiozen an official test. But the Food and Drug Administration never approved the substance for sale.

America's romance with Laetrile constitutes a fascinating story of the relation between science and politics. Prepared from apricot pits, the drug—known generically as amygdalin—had been used since ancient times for a variety of illnesses and had been widely used in the United States since the 1920s. The trade name "Laetrile" was introduced by Ernest Krebs, Jr., who obtained a United States patent for it in 1952; and it attained great popularity in the 1960s and 1970s. The Food and Drug Administration rejected requests for its licensure, but twenty-seven states permitted its sale. A 1977 Harris poll indicated overwhelming support among the American public for its legalization. Over 50,000 cancer patients were reported to have taken the drug in that year.[34] Supporters pressed for legalization at the federal level, or at least a clinical trial by the National Institutes of Health.

The medical and scientific communities experienced strong crosscurrents in the legalization controversy. Most medical organizations opposed legalization. Leading medical researchers objected that in the absence of animal experiments it would be unethical even to test the drug on human subjects. Some expressed special alarm at the thought that the conduct of a test would signal the replacement of scientific neutrality by politics in the setting of research priorities. However, many individual physicians seemed to accommodate legalization and warmed to the idea of a clinical trial. These supporters argued that legalization would relieve patients in states where the drug was not sold from having to procure it underground, thereby seeking care from nonphysicians. According to this reasoning, the patient who obtained Laetrile from a physician would be more likely to undergo standard care along with the unorthodox medication. Still others, noting the appearance of contaminated Laetrile in the underground market, reasoned that legalization would allow the drug to be produced and distributed under pharmaceutically controlled conditions.

The National Cancer Institute finally sponsored a clinical trial of Laetrile in the early 1980s. The comments of Dr. Charles Moertel of the Mayo Clinic, the research team leader, acknowledge the conflicting forces that led to the study:

Whereas [evidence for the effectiveness of Laetrile] can be challenged, of greater concern is the fact that Laetrile has remained a major and unresolved public health problem for over a quarter of a century, involving many thousands of cancer patients in direct treatment and causing serious doubts and concerns in many more. In addition, a valid scientific question could be raised if this widespread and continued public acceptance possibly reflected true therapeutic activity, animal-model data nonwithstanding. These humanitarian and scientific issues were the primary considerations that led to National Cancer Institute sponsorship and Food and Drug Administration approval of a clinical trial of amygdalin for the treatment of advanced cancer.[35]

The actual clinical trial of Laetrile included 179 patients with advanced cancer, for which no treatments existed that could be expected to cure the disease or extend life. Most patients were given Laetrile in doses considered appropriate by practitioners in the community who prescribed Laetrile; these patients also received "metabolic therapy," the large doses of vitamins and pancreatic enzyme that often accompanied standard Laetrile treatment. A small subgroup received higher doses of Laetrile, as well as the metabolic treatment.

Medical journals have reported few clinical trials with clearer results than Moertel's Laetrile study. Only one patient showed any sign of tumor response. Within eighteen months of treatment, 152 of the patients died. The study indicated, moreover, that patients who took Laetrile risked arsenic poisoning from traces found in natural amygdalin.[36]

The 1970s and 1980s saw popularization of a second unorthodox cancer treatment with support from the very prominent. Nobel laureate Linus Pauling became a leading advocate for vitamin C treatments. Vitamin C enjoyed several great advantages over Laetrile in gaining popularity among cancer patients. It could be taken orally. Some animal studies and test-tube experiments supported the potential value of vitamin C in cancer. Furthermore, being a vitamin, it could be purchased over the counter, not requiring Food and Drug Administration approval. Vitamin C became one of the most widely used alternative cancer treatments.

The federal government sponsored two clinical investigations of vitamin C as a treatment for advanced cancer. Both studies were double blind; that is, neither the subjects nor the investigators knew who was in the experimental group and who was a control. The first trial compared two groups of patients with advanced cancer. One group (sixty patients) received high doses of vitamin C; the other group (sixty-three patients) received a flavored sugar pill. The vitamin C and the sugar placebo were given in identical capsules. Within thirty-two weeks, nearly all these patients had died. Those who took the sugar pills and the vitamin C survived identical lengths of time.[37]

Unconvinced, Pauling objected that the research team, again including the Mayo Clinic's Dr. Moertel, had performed their experiment on an inappropriate group of patients. Pauling argued that many of these patients had received chemotherapy prior to the vitamin C trial. Chemotherapy, he asserted, could have damaged the patients' immune systems and rendered the vitamin C intervention useless. Moertel and his colleagues conducted a second trial, this time excluding patients who had received chemotherapy. In this study, the investigators found not only that patients taking vitamin C obtained no apparent advantage but also that those who took the sugar pills tended to live *longer*.[38] Pauling continued to object that the clinical trials were flawed; he remained an active advocate for vitamin C.[39]

To many scientists and physicians, the widespread use of alternative therapies may appear repugnant and shocking. But the practice cannot be attributed to ignorance or desperation. A fascinating study of unorthodox treatment methods, published in 1984, revealed that 13 percent of patients receiving care at a major medical center reported using some form of alternative therapy. Of those receiving alternative treatment, 42 percent had localized disease; *higher* levels of education tended to correspond with unorthodox therapies. Most of those receiving alternative treatments also received conventional care; physicians holding M.D. degrees delivered much of this care or referred their patients to alternative practitioners.[40]

Seeking therapies outside conventional medicine had not become old-fashioned in the late twentieth century. Patients appeared to seek this form of care in order to experience more direct control over their lives at a time when conventional medicine offered them only passive roles in the treatment effort. It seems likely that these patients derived emotional gratification from the process of alternative treatment. But if Krebiozen, Laetrile, and megadoses of vitamin C were representative, these patients obtained no advantage whatsoever in the search for cure.

The World of Cancer Science

Most people in modern America believe in science. When they think of a research laboratory, most Americans visualize men and women dedicating their lives to the single-minded pursuit of discovery. If there is any professional setting where deliberate, rational thinking replaces fashion and prejudice, it is expected to be cancer research. If there is any human endeavor where men and women abandon personal ambition and cynicism, it is assumed to be in the search for causes and cures of cancer, the scourge of modern humankind. The citizen, however, must develop a more realistic view of this important segment of "the industry of hope" in order to ask appropriate questions about the claims of cancer researchers.

It is important to realize that cancer research is a highly competitive field, where major investigators struggle constantly to obtain funds for large research projects. As technology progressed throughout the century, research became increasingly expensive and research teams grew substantially in size. When prominent investigator Robert A. Good, for example, joined the Memorial Sloan-Kettering Institute as director of cancer research, he brought fifty junior investigators with him. In the 1980s and 1990s, however, individual biomedical scientists found it increasingly difficult to obtain support as more and more competed for a decreasing number of grants.

In this scramble for resources, top scientists must function as highly sophisticated advocates for the type of cancer research in which they exercise leadership. In this role, they must socialize with the boards of trustees of major research institutions, control important journals, and participate in government panels. They may also do important services for people whose wealth and power they need to keep their laboratories open. As one observer has written,

Philanthropy has funded much research in universities. Families who have given money to these programs often expect both personal and societal benefits to result from their support. An objective review of programs in universities would clearly show that "funding fathers" receive special attention and often special care. Few would suggest that such philanthropic funding be discontinued because everyone does not have access to a special effort made by the university medical faculty on behalf of donors when those philanthropists, or their relatives or friends, are in need.[41]

Junior scientists feel tremendous pressure to demonstrate visible success in this atmosphere of competition. Scientific papers must be published constantly, and progress must be continuously demonstrated; otherwise, research funds and jobs may be lost. Men and women remain in their laboratories far into the night. For at least a few, the pressure to produce has encouraged fabrication of research results. A review published by the *New York Times* indicated that scientific fraud had occurred at Sloan-Kettering and Yale, Cornell, Harvard, and Boston Universities during the 1980s.[42] In 1983, the National Institutes of Health sent a bill to Harvard Medical School, seeking restitution of $122,000 for a faked series of experiments. Scientific fraud seems to occur in part because senior scientists can no longer keep track of their large projects. Of his superior, a junior investigator at Sloan-Kettering who forged research results remarked, "It was often hard to get to talk to him. . . . I used to get up at four or five o'clock in the morning to see him for a few minutes."

Both the prestige and the technical complexity of science have created major barriers to public oversight of the research enterprise. In one of the late twentieth century's most celebrated examples of this phenomenon, the powerful congressman John D. Dingell and the Nobel laureate David Baltimore confronted each other during an investigation of scientific fraud and misconduct. Defending a colleague against the charge of data-faking in the 1980s, Baltimore charged that the congressional investigation led by Dingell gave scientists the message that they should carry out their research "with an eye toward facing prosecution on the style" of their science. Press accounts included terms such as *witch hunt* and *Galileo trial*.[43] A 1991 report by the National Institutes of Health, however, confirmed that data falsification had indeed taken place over several years, fraudulent results had appeared in a prestigious scientific journal, and a whistle-blower had been fired from the laboratory in which the misconduct allegedly took place.[44] Fearing that the case would appear to prove the scientific community's ability to "cover up the errors of eminent insiders," a prominent journal editor criticized Baltimore for brushing aside valid criticism "as much from overconfidence as from loyalty" to his colleague.[45]

Exaggerated reports of cancer "breakthroughs" regularly appear in the mass media. Individual scientists may exercise restraint in talking with the press. But the strength of the public's desire for a cancer cure tempts researcher and reporter alike to overlook the problems in a study and the complexity of its findings. A drug company holding rights to a new treatment has a strong incentive to see that research results are presented in the most favorable light possible. By 1990, it should be noted, for-profit drug and biotechnology companies funded a very high proportion of the medical research taking place in the United States.

Critics have questioned the research establishment's commitment to full exploration of scientific leads. Major shifts in emphasis in cancer research have regularly taken place since the 1940s, when the enterprise first received serious funding. Areas in fashion have included metabolism, endocrinology, virology, chemotherapy, chemoprevention, and immunology, to name only a few. To what degree these shifts reflect frustration with scientific blind alleys or simply mirror turnovers in political battles among scientists remains an open question.

Physicians seem to recognize the limitations of research. A 1986 study of 118 Canadian physicians asked whether they would participate as patients in several hypothetical clinical trials for non–small cell lung cancer. The hypothetical descriptions paralleled actual clinical trials taking place at that time. All the physicians questioned were specialists in lung cancer treatment. Clear majorities of these physicians said they would not participate in several of the trials, which involved chemotherapy or radiation. Those who said they would refuse explained that they did not think chemotherapy or radiation would be effective against this disease and that the interventions would cause serious side effects. The authors of the study conclude, "the finding that most specialists who treat lung cancer would not consent to participate as subjects in many of these trials is of concern. If experts refuse to participate in a trial, should uncomprehending patients be asked to consent?"[46]

◆   ◆   ◆   ◆   ◆

Cancer treatment today makes increased survival possible for a large number of Americans. For most, the greatest benefits will come in the form of well-tested, skillfully applied, conventional care. Experimental treatment, while important for the progress of science, offers little hope of greatly extending the life span of most patients who participate in clinical trials. Under objective scrutiny, alternative treatments offer no benefits in the form of increased survival.

It appears, then, that the best way to reduce cancer deaths is to promote timely access to conventional care. But many scientists and laypeople argue for approaches that do not rely primarily on conventional treatment. Some assert that many if not most cancers can be prevented and that, therefore, new efforts to reduce the threat to life represented by cancer should address not treatment but prevention. Others contend that emotional well-being has a strong impact on cancer survival and that, therefore, health care must begin to shift emphasis toward psychological interventions aimed at favorably altering the patient's outlook and mood—certainly a departure from the basic approach of conventional treatment. The importance of conventional medical care can be estimated only after the potential contributions of prevention and psychological interventions have been assessed.

Prevention moved to center stage in the increasingly health-conscious America of the late twentieth century. How much cancer can, in fact, be prevented? An answer to this question can lead to development of an appropriate balance of prevention and treatment in efforts to improve cancer survival.

CHAPTER FOUR

Can Cancer Be Prevented?

Compared with the era when science conquered infectious disease, historians will probably find the late twentieth century unremarkable. As the century draws to a close, Americans face an increasing risk of death from cancer. The long view, covering the development of modern medicine since 1900, reveals significant progress. But in the 1990s, science and medicine did not seem poised for breakthroughs. Exciting reports about revolutionary cures often proved unfounded. Perhaps in frustration, many people began looking toward prevention.

Prevention makes sense. As the preceding chapters demonstrate, physicians cannot usually cure many forms of cancer. If a high proportion of cancers can, in fact, be prevented, many people may avert the *threat* that cancer represents, obviating the issue of survival. Large-scale cancer prevention could mean reduction of America's vast and costly anticancer armory of health care professionals, hospitals, radiation machines, drugs, and scalpels. For the individual, strong ties with the medical care system would become less necessary. For the policymaker, the issue of access to medical care would become less acute.

This chapter assesses the effectiveness of cancer prevention. It asks how much of the past century's reliance on cure can be replaced by prevention in the century to come. Perhaps the lives we live, the air we breathe, the foods we eat hold the key to cancer. In the thinking of many, a revolution in ecological consciousness and lifestyle appears more likely to reduce the threat of cancer than would a revolution in the research laboratory.

Exogenous Causes of Cancer: Opportunities for Prevention

Effective cancer prevention requires recognition of *exogenous* causes of the disease—factors that originate outside the body. Some experts, in fact, prefer to characterize these factors simply as "environmental." The exogenous causes of cancer include a large number of agents and stimuli recognizable above the level of the cellular changes that initiate malignant disease. Phenomena of this kind are presumably more easily recognizable than those lurking in the deep recesses of cells. Once recognized, it is thought, they can be controlled.

Physicians and scientists have recognized exogenous causes of cancer for hundreds of years. Discovery of such factors often began as an observation that some people, particularly those in certain trades or professions, have especially high risks of developing cancer. Exposure to hazards at the workplace, such as industrial chemicals, has presented the most obvious risk. Modern observers have included radiation, diet, and personal lifestyle practices in this area of concern, expanding the notions of "exogenous" and "environmental" beyond their original meanings.

Exogenous stimuli appear to cause or contribute to the *initiation* of cancer by damaging the structure of DNA in the cell. An exogenous stimulus may also *promote* the proliferation of cancer cells and the development of tumors by helping create conditions within the body that are favorable to cancer growth. One exogenous factor may have its most powerful effect when combined with another, the two multiplying each other's influence.

Exogenous causes of cancer, proven and suspected, became public issues in the 1960s and 1970s, surfacing alongside more general concerns with ecology and the environment. Chemical hazards and pollution attracted the widest attention. In 1967, one authority estimated that 90 percent of cancers were caused by chemicals in the environment.[1] A highly comprehensive analysis, examining chemicals (mostly industrial exposure), radiation, diet, alcohol, and tobacco, concluded that "in most parts of the United States in 1970 about 75 or 80 percent of the cases of cancer in both sexes might have been avoidable."[2]

These and other estimates have led to a widespread belief among both laypeople and health professionals that most cancers are environmental in origin. A strong tradition of research has indeed identified many exogenous factors as causes of cancer. But the conclusion that most cancer is avoidable is so striking that the related research requires very careful examination. Assessment of the degree to which prevention can actually replace cure requires weighing the evidence. Risks associated with chemicals, lifestyle, and other exogenous causes of cancer must be systematically compared with those that unquestionably reside, in varying degrees, within the organs, tissues, and cells of every human being.

HAZARDOUS SUBSTANCES AND CHEMICALS

The late twentieth century brought widespread awareness in the minds of the public and health professionals that exposure to the by-products of industrial development increased the individual's likelihood of contracting cancer. Many industrial processes utilize or produce carcinogenic substances to which workers face potential exposure. People with no industrial exposure face similar hazards, as suspect chemicals are released into the atmosphere and water supply, remain active as manufactured products, or are produced by consumers themselves.

Astute observers of public health have realized the connection between hazardous substances and cancer for centuries. As long ago as the 1500s, observers linked exposure to arsenic with skin disease. In the twentieth century, researchers demonstrated that people exposed to arsenic in the metal-smelting industry or through air and water pollution tended to develop cancers of the lung and skin. In the 1700s, the English surgeon Sir Percival Pott noticed that chimney sweeps had a surprisingly high probability of developing cancer of the scrotum. Progress in the techniques available to science and medicine allowed twentieth-century investigators to link scrotal cancer to a specific chemical found in coal tar (benzopyrene).

The period between the late 1800s and the mid-twentieth century brought a rapid succession of discoveries linking industrial chemicals and cancer. Milestones included discovery of a link between organic chemicals used in the German dye industry and bladder cancer (1895); between chromates and lung cancer in miners and smelters (1948); between asbestos and a variety of cancers in several industries (1949).[3]

Inaction by industrialists or public officials in response to long-recognized hazards has produced outrage among some public health spokespersons. As long ago as the 1800s, life insurance companies noted the high rate of early deaths among workers in locomotive shops, where much asbestos was used, and refused them coverage. Yet asbestos remained in widespread use through most of the twentieth century. Thousands received massive exposure to asbestos with minimal protection in the shipyards of World War II. Millions completely outside asbestos-related industries received doses of asbestos through its use in the construction of homes, schools, hospitals, roads, and recreational facilities, or its presence in food, water, and air. A crusade by Dr. Irving Selikoff and others in the 1960s and 1970s finally mobilized organized labor and the public health profession to safeguard asbestos workers and remove asbestos from the environment.

By the late twentieth century, scientists were taking more proactive steps to identify cancer-causing substances. One method, rodent bioassay, simply exposed laboratory mice and rats to high concentrations of the suspected substance and observed the animals over their lifetimes to determine whether cancers developed. Because rodent bioassay was expensive and time-consuming, scientists developed an alternative method, called "mutagenesis assay," for testing suspected cancer-causing agents. This type of test makes use of the fact that cancer-causing chemicals usually have their strongest effects in the initiation phase of cancer development. Typically, these agents cause cancer by damaging DNA, resulting in production of abnormal cells. In mutagenesis assay, investigators expose well-known strains of bacteria to the substance suspected of causing cancer, and look for signs that the exposure gives rise to mutant cells.[4] If mutant cells do appear, the suspect chemical is subjected to further testing.

Even the development of actual cancer in rodents does not indicate that a chemical causes cancer in humans. Such a conclusion would require epidemiological validation, based on comparison of cancer rates among people exposed to the suspected agent and those without such exposure. At least in the modern United States, scientists do not purposely expose people to suspected chemicals to see whether they cause cancer. They may, however, keep track of people who work in industries that produce, utilize, or otherwise promote exposure to suspect chemicals. The experience of workers in such industries generates knowledge about substances with which citizens and consumers may come in contact regularly, although in weaker concentrations.

By the 1980s, scientists had accumulated solid evidence that workers in a small number of industries faced heightened risks of cancer, which could be traced to specific chemicals and processes. A landmark review by the English scientists Richard Doll and Robert Peto of all research completed by 1980 serves as an excellent source of information in this crucial area.[5] Miners and metal refiners face a variety of cancer risks as a result of chemical exposure. Copper and cobalt smelters have elevated risks of skin and lung cancer because of contact with arsenic, a hazard shared by some pesticide manufacturers. Cadmium workers have higher rates of prostate cancer because of their exposure to the metal. Chromium workers, including people who manufacture paints containing chromium, have high rates of lung cancer. Nickel refiners have an elevated tendency to contract nasal, sinus, and lung cancers.

In other industries, complex organic chemicals—particularly polycyclic hydrocarbons, elaborate chains and rings of carbon atoms—have been found to cause cancer. Persons employed in dye and rubber manufacturing may be exposed to a class of chemicals called aromatic amines, which cause bladder cancer. Workers exposed to benzene in the manufacture of glues and varnishes may contract blood-related cancers. Persons who work with coal tar derivatives—for instance, gas workers, roofers, asphalters, and aluminum refiners—have a tendency to develop cancers of the skin, scrotum, and lung. Vinyl chloride causes cancer of the liver and nasal sinuses among workers who manufacture this widely used substance, as well as among hardwood furniture makers and leather workers, who use it in their industries.

According to Doll and Peto, cancer-causing chemicals and processes encountered in industry accounted for about 4 percent of all cancer deaths in the United States in 1978. Taking into account both the potency of the agents involved and the number of people affected, they concluded that the greatest threats occurred in lung and bladder cancer and leukemia. These researchers estimated that industrial hazards caused 15 percent of the deaths from lung cancer, 10 percent of the deaths from bladder cancer, and 10 percent of the deaths from leukemia. Radiation, which may cause leukemia and which sometimes occurs as an industrial hazard, receives detailed attention below.

People who work outside the industries described above face hazards related to some of the same substances, which are distributed as components of consumer goods or are purposely or accidentally released into the environment. Asbestos used in construction and some consumer goods represents a continuing threat. Cancer has been linked with a variety of pesticides, including DDT and the grain fumigant EDB (ethylene dibromide).[6] While workers involved in the manufacture or utilization of these chemicals encounter higher doses, others may take in their residues with food.

RADIATION

"Radiation" joins "hazardous chemicals" as a major scare word related to cancer. The term *radiation* generally refers to energy emitted from a source in the form of particles or waves. All radiation transmits energy from its source to a target: radio waves from an oscillating electrical circuit, radar beams from a radar transmitter, light from an incandescent filament. The level of energy associated with a particular form of radiation is measured by its frequency and wavelength. Higher frequency and shorter wavelength correspond to greater energy. The range of energy levels in various kinds of radiation is called the electromagnetic spectrum, encompassing, in order of increasing energy, radio waves, microwaves, infrared light, visible light, ultraviolet light, and ionizing radiation. Ionizing radiation, with sufficient energy to knock electrons out of their atomic orbits, encompasses X rays, alpha and beta particles, gamma rays, and, at the far end of the spectrum, cosmic rays. Ultraviolet light and all ionizing radiation are known to cause cancer.

Like hazardous chemicals, ionizing radiation may damage the structure of DNA required for normal cell reproduction. When high-energy particles or rays strike individual cells, they impart energy to its molecules, including the DNA. Many scientists adhere to the so-called two-hit theory, believing that radiation must affect at least two very nearby cells to produce visible tissue abnormality.[7] This logic suggests that greater radiation exposure will result in more tissue damage and an increased possibility of cancer. Certain kinds of ultraviolet light may also induce changes in DNA.[8]

Like hazardous chemicals, radiation has become a major public concern. Part of this concern has arisen from the belief that officials in government and industry, while aware of the risks represented by radiation, kept this information secret. The comments of Dr. H. Jack Geiger, a professor of community medicine and prominent public health spokesperson, exemplify this concern. With reference to the Hanford facility in Washington, operated since World War II for nuclear weapons research and manufacture, Geiger wrote in 1990:

Never have so many human beings been exposed to so much radiation over so long a time—while so few knew about it. Now, more than 40 years after it began, we are just beginning to learn what the U.S. government's Hanford nuclear weapons plant in Washington State has done to thousands of citizens who unwittingly drank radioactively contaminated water, breathed radioactively contaminated air, and fed milk laced with radioactive iodine to their children. . . . From 1944 to 1947 alone, the nuclear weapons factory spewed 400,000 curies of radioactive iodine into the atmosphere. The bodily absorption of 50 millionths of a single curie is sufficient to raise the risk of thyroid cancer. For years thereafter, Hanford poured radioactive water into the Columbia River, and leaked millions of gallons of radioactive waste from damaged tanks into the groundwater.

Geiger charged the "Department of Energy, its predecessor agencies and their contractors" with an "official coverup," "two decades of lies," and "callous indifference to public health."[9]

Potentially cancer-causing radiation comes from many less sensational sources than the Hanford plant. Since the 1800s, medical and scientific reports have noted high rates of skin cancer among people such as farmers and sailors exposed to large amounts of sunshine. Several forms of skin cancer are relatively harmless, not spreading very far beyond their origins and easily removable by surgery. Malignant melanoma, however, which comprises about 5 percent of all skin cancers, was estimated to cause 6,300 deaths in the United States in 1990.[10]

Ultraviolet light is the cancer-causing agent in sunshine. Fair-skinned people living in desert areas or southern latitudes face the highest risks of contracting skin cancer. Data collected around 1970 illustrate the effect of sunlight on these risks. White people living in Fort Worth, Texas, had well over twice the risk of developing malignant melanoma as those in Minneapolis, Minnesota. Fort Worth is located at 32.8 degrees north latitude and receives twice as much ultraviolet radiation as Minneapolis at 44.9 degrees north.[11]

Ionizing radiation is more powerful than sunlight as a cause of cancer. Workers in industries that utilize radioactive materials experience elevated risks of cancer. Medical and dental procedures expose patients to radiation. People near the sites of atomic and hydrogen bomb detonations have absorbed significant amounts of radiation in their bodies. The natural environment itself contains many sources of radiation. In addition to sunlight, naturally occurring radioactive material in the earth heightens cancer risks. Cosmic radiation from outer space contributes significantly to the incidence of cancer.

Workers in industries that utilize radioactive materials have been the subject of intense interest. A classic investigation of women employed in the radium dial–painting industry before 1930 revealed a high incidence of bone cancer.[12] In order to keep their points fine, workers often licked the brushes they used to paint the dials of watches and clocks. This practice resulted in actual ingestion of the radium. A study of uranium miners indicates that they are over five times as likely as the general population to develop respiratory cancers.[13] Security regulations prohibited independent scientists from obtaining data on the health of workers at nuclear facilities such as Hanford for most of the twentieth century. Studies based on these data were not yet available at the time this book was written.

Physicians and dentists must share the blame for many avoidable cancers. The history of medicine before the late twentieth century was marked by extensive overuse of radiation. Doctors used X rays to treat rheumatoid conditions, enlarged thymus glands, ringworm, and tonsil ailments. These procedures resulted in elevated rates of cancer in the organs targeted for medical treatment and in anatomical sites in the path of the radiation beams.[14] Growing awareness of the hazards represented by radiation led medicine to abandon many of these practices around mid-century. Physicians and dentists, of course, still use X rays and other radiation-dependent imaging techniques to help diagnose illnesses and injuries. These techniques have become considerably safer over the years because equipment now focuses X-ray beams more precisely and films require less exposure time.

Still, the use of radiation-based diagnostic tools—even such techniques as mammography, designed to provide early detection of breast cancer—involves some cancer risk. One investigator has identified medical procedures as the source of the greatest average radiation exposure for the United States population. He indicates that people who undergo medical procedures involving radiation receive an average dose of 120 millirems (a measure of radiation absorbed by the body). In comparison, the average worker at a nuclear power plant receives a dose of 400 millirems—higher, but within the same general range.[15]

Populations near the detonation sites of atomic and hydrogen bombs received high doses of radiation from the blasts themselves and from subsequent fallout. The continuing study of persons who survived the atomic bombings of Hiroshima and Nagasaki in 1945 must serve as one of the key documents of the nuclear age. Increased rates of leukemia, which were most marked among young children, became apparent one year after the bombing. The risk of leukemia continued to rise for six to seven years after the bombing, and then declined steadily. Forty-three years after the bombing, leukemia deaths among those exposed to intense radiation were more than double the leukemia deaths among those not exposed. Deaths from other cancers also increased, though at a lesser rate, including cancers of the stomach, colon, lung, breast, urinary tract, and bone marrow.[16]

Exposure to radioactive fallout also increases cancer risks, although to a much lesser degree. Two hundred residents of the Marshall Islands who were exposed to fallout from a United States hydrogen bomb test in 1954 were examined regularly for twenty years. Girls (but not boys or adults of either sex) developed thyroid cancers in unexpectedly high numbers.[17] Military personnel present at a famous Nevada nuclear detonation called "Smoky" experienced an increased risk of leukemia—exposed soldiers developed leukemia at over twice the rate normally expected.[18] Among children growing up in Utah during the era of aboveground bomb testing, fallout exposure was weakly related to death from leukemia. According to a highly regarded study led by Dr. Walter Stevens of the University of Utah, the relationship between exposure to fallout and death from leukemia was so small that it could have been observed purely by chance.[19]

Natural sources of radiation include soil, rocks, food, and water that contain naturally occurring radioactive elements, as well as cosmic rays. People living in Denver experience higher radiation exposure than those at sea level because of their greater exposure to cosmic rays. It is estimated that 50 percent of radiation exposure to the United States population comes from natural sources. According to one investigator, natural background radiation accounts for an average dose in the United States population of 80 millirems, compared with an average of 3 millirems for airline travelers and about 1 millirem for those who live near (but do not work in) nuclear power plants.[20]

Radon, an inert, radioactive gas occurring naturally in the soil, has drawn significant attention in the parts of the United States where it is common—for instance, in certain areas of the Northeast. This gas seeps into houses, giving rise over time to radioactive compounds. A lifetime of breathing radon at levels often found in the home produces a lung cancer risk of 1 per 1,000, in the absence of other risk factors. Between 0.5 and 2.0 percent of U.S. homes have radon levels eight times the normal level, raising the risk of lung cancer to 16 per 1,000.[21]

Public concern has arisen in recent years over the possibility that still other forms of radiation may cause cancer. High-tension power lines produce electromagnetic fields, which, according to some, can cause leukemia. Studies of this form of radiation, whose energy level is too low to cause ionization, have not produced any clear indication of danger.[22] A large study, involving 20,000 Navy radar technicians who performed tasks associated with microwave radiation, found no increase in the risk of cancer.[23] Computer programmers, word processors, and others who work at cathode-ray terminals (CRTs) have become concerned that radiation from these devices exposes them to cancer risk. CRTs are essentially television screens, which do emit some ionizing radiation. The amount of radiation an average American absorbs per year from television viewing is about .5 millirem—small in comparison with the annual radiation exposure of the average airline traveler, and tiny in comparison with natural background radiation.

DIET

Most health professionals and an ever larger segment of the public recognize the importance of diet in the maintenance of good health. Health authorities were joined by gurus and cultists of all kinds in the late twentieth century in urging the adoption of specialized food regimens. The death of nutrition spokesperson Adele Davis from cancer at a not especially old age in the 1970s may have weakened the dietary commitments of some. But, while perhaps exaggerated in some quarters, diet has real importance in prevention of illness. Substantial research suggests that diet affects cancer risk.

Food Additives. "Poison in the food" always attracts attention. Throughout the late twentieth century, the news media carried stories about newly discovered cancer risks from chemicals widely used in the flavoring, coloration, or preservation of food. Alleged danger from food additives has always made good copy. But there is little or no scientific evidence that food additives pose significant, widespread cancer risks.

Today food additives undergo careful laboratory screening. Before such testing was routinely performed, some chemicals later found to cause cancer were widely used. A cancer-causing chemical dye called "butter yellow," for example, was used for many years to make margarine look like the real thing. The additive is no longer used for this purpose. The most intense discussion in the United States during this era focused on saccharin, a ubiquitous sweetener invented in 1902, and nitrites, a class of chemicals long used to preserve and flavor meats. Saccharin and nitrites have been regularly ingested by millions of people.

Several widely used artificial sweeteners were legally banned as food additives in 1968. Federal legislation a decade earlier had required the U.S. Food and Drug Administration to ban all food additives that had been found to cause cancer in human beings or animals. Rats fed and injected with large quantities of saccharin had been shown to develop bladder cancer.

The rat study, however, did not demonstrate that saccharin could cause cancer in human beings. It is practically impossible to imagine a human taking in as much saccharin per body weight as the laboratory rats had received. Other species of laboratory animals, including mice, hamsters, and monkeys, did not develop cancer when fed large quantities of saccharin. The United States experienced no major increase in bladder cancer after the introduction of saccharin; diabetics, more likely to use sugar substitutes such as saccharin and cyclamates than others, evidenced no proclivity to contracting cancer.[24]

Evidence linking nitrites in food with cancer in humans proved to be even weaker. Experiments with animals indicate that ingested nitrites react with other substances derived from food, as well as digestive juices, to form carcinogenic compounds in the body.[25] In rodents and other animals, the compounds derived from nitrites have caused cancers of the liver, kidney, esophagus, and respiratory tract.[26] But serious doubts remained about whether nitrites taken in with food significantly contributed to the formation of carcinogens in the body. No scientific consensus ever developed about the degree of risk (if any) that people incurred when they ate meat or other foods prepared or preserved with nitrites. While public concern was aroused and "aware" individuals may have avoided them, nitrites were never banned.

Dietary Fat. Perhaps no other food component has received as much attention as fat. Most people know that a diet high in fats can lead to impaired blood circulation, causing heart attacks and strokes. The effects of fatty foods on personal appearance have doubtless contributed to the widespread belief that they are deleterious to health. Certainly, research has identified body weight as a contributor to heart attacks, strokes, and other life-threatening illnesses. More recently, scientists have uncovered evidence that a diet containing too much fatty food can also cause cancer.

Scientists who believe that a connection exists between fatty foods and cancer have several powerful theories to support their thinking. One of the major theories focuses on the promotion phase of cancer development, during which changes in body chemistry stimulate a few abnormal cells to multiply. Researchers have reported that fatty substances in the diet give rise to high levels of the hormones that promote development of tumors. All things being equal, people who consume a fatty diet risk becoming overweight, their weight gain coming primarily from an increase of fat (adipose) tissue. An important study has demonstrated that an enzyme in human fat tissue enables the body to produce an especially potent hormone.[27] This and related hormones, it is believed, create an environment in the body that encourages the tiny number of abnormal cells which may exist to multiply and form visible tumors.[28]

Researchers have demonstrated that fat people face especially high risks of cancer. A massive study by the American Cancer Society in the 1970s, which followed 750,000 people for thirteen years, demonstrated that the overweight were much more likely to die from cancer than people in the normal weight range. Women whose weight was 40 percent above normal, for example, had five times as high a rate of death from endometrial cancer and twice as high a rate from cervical cancer as those of normal weight. Men whose weight was 40 percent above normal had a 70 percent greater chance of dying from colon cancer and a 30 percent greater chance of dying from prostate cancer.[29] Other studies reported even stronger relationships between overweight and dying from some forms of cancer.

Not all scientists believe that hormones associated with fat promote cancer development.[30] But some scientists have developed explanations that do not involve hormones as intervening factors in the linkage between fatty diets and cancer. These researchers focus on colon cancer and the effects of dietary fat on bowel contents. In a series of research studies beginning in the 1960s, scientists have examined the feces of population groups throughout the world, comparing those that have high rates of colon cancer with those having low rates.[31] These comparisons have revealed that groups whose diets were high in fats had high concentrations in their large intestines of certain steroids, bile acids, and microorganisms. Members of these groups were the very ones who faced the highest risks of contracting cancer of the colon. Ongoing research in this area proved inconclusive, however—some studies continuing to demonstrate a relation between eating fat and developing colon cancer, others turning out neutral or contradictory.[32]

Nobody really knows why some groups that have little fat in their diets are less likely to develop cancer. Reports in this area tend to identify total dietary fat as the culprit. Attempts to find relationships with more specific dietary components and their products have not been successful. Meat eating (except for fats contained in many meats) does not seem to be related to malignancies. Serum cholesterol, important in the development of heart disease, has not been isolated as a cause of cancer.

In the late twentieth century, researchers characterized some forms of cancer as "diseases of the affluent." Colon and breast cancer, for example, seemed to strike the city dweller who had sufficient resources to consume processed foods, meats, and other fat-containing items more often than the peasant who obtained his or her nutrition from grains and other traditional sources. A comparison of Japanese-Americans living in Hawaii in the 1970s with both Hawaiian Caucasians and Japanese living in Japan seems to support this general impression. Among the Japanese-Americans living in Hawaii, rates of colon and breast cancer more closely approximated those of the Caucasian population than those prevailing in Japan.[33] It is tempting to infer that the Japanese-Americans in Hawaii, mostly descendants of immigrants in earlier generations, had adopted the food habits (including increased fat consumption) of their Caucasian neighbors, and thus incurred similar cancer risks.

Beta-Carotene and Vitamin A. The possibility that vitamin A and substances related to it prevent cancer has caused great excitement in medical and public health circles. Interest has focused principally on beta-carotene. Found in green and yellow vegetables (especially, of course, in carrots), fruits, and other foods of plant origin, beta-carotene is converted to vitamin A in the intestines. In the 1970s, researchers began to suspect that beta-carotene inhibited the promotion of cancer within the body. Although abnormal cells may have already been present, the theory went, beta-carotene kept them from developing into truly malignant cells and proliferating to become visible tumors. Evidence for this theory began to accumulate from studies using experimental animals and cell cultures.

Several large-scale, long-term studies concluded in the 1970s and 1980s indicated relationships between vitamin A (and related substances) and reduced risk of lung cancer in humans. A five-year study of over 8,000 Norwegian men indicated that those whose diet included larger amounts of foods containing (or capable of producing) vitamin A experienced lower risks of lung cancer. Reduced occurrence of lung cancer was found even among cigarette smokers. This finding was confirmed by studies of thousands of additional individuals in the United States, Singapore, and Japan. Two important studies saved and analyzed blood samples from apparently healthy people in Maryland and Japan. Those who developed lung cancer in later years were found to have had relatively low levels of beta-carotene in their blood serum. Still other studies have reported a preventive effect of beta-carotene on several forms of cancer other than lung.[34]

Like other lines of inquiry on dietary practices and cancer, studies of beta-carotene and cancer have not produced entirely consistent results. After reviewing seven well-conducted studies carried out in the 1980s, one authority concluded that "those in the lowest third to quarter of the population distribution of carotene intake" had between a 50 and 100 percent greater risk of lung cancer.[35] Other studies, however, which examined *all* forms of cancer, found no evidence that beta-carotene or vitamin A helped protect against malignancies.[36] Researchers in the 1990s, moreover, were still not sure whether vitamin A, beta-carotene, some other carotene-related substance, or a constituent of fruits and vegetables unrelated to any of these accounted for the observations of a preventive effect.

Fiber. In the 1980s, messages to the public about the advantages of dietary fiber became frequent. Some research offered support for the belief that high amounts of fiber in the diet could help prevent cancer of the colon, one of the most widespread forms of cancer in the United States. The American Cancer Society recommended that Americans "eat more high-fiber foods such as whole grain cereals, fruits, and vegetables" to "help reduce the risk of colon cancer." The cautious advice of the American Cancer Society became a highly visible marketing message in the hands of food manufacturers, who highlighted the connection between fiber and cancer prevention in their packaging and promotion of cereals and baked goods of all kinds. "Fiber" became a household word, its role in preventing cancer the kind of health fact that "everybody knows."

Yet scientists have trouble agreeing on many things about fiber. First, what is it? An early investigator of the effects of fiber on cancer risks defined it as the components of plant cell walls that resist digestion in the human body. This definition includes a broad range of substances that may be found in food. Other scientists have included an even broader range of substances: undigestible or partially digestible proteins, sugars, and starches; cellulose; gums; mucilages; shell material from shrimp and other crustaceans; waxes; silicon.[37] Clearly, substantial differences exist among these substances. Some are composed of relatively simple molecules; others, highly complex ones. Some dissolve in water; others do not. Some are almost entirely digested in human intestines; others pass through largely unaffected by human digestive agents.

The most important theory attributing an important role to dietary fiber in the prevention of colon cancer rests on the presumption that this substance absorbs or dilutes acids, biles, and other potential carcinogens in the large intestine, reducing their effects in initiating or promoting cancer. It is also thought that high levels of dietary fiber decrease the "transit time" of feces—that is, the time which passes between eating and excreting—and thus reduce the period during which carcinogens are in contact with intestinal tissues.

Several early studies demonstrated relationships between high dietary fiber and low rates of colon cancer. One representative study published in 1977 compared residents of Copenhagen, Denmark, and Kuopio, Finland. Although people in both locations consumed similar amounts of several nutrients, including fat, those in Kuopio consumed significantly higher amounts of fiber. Colon cancer was four times as frequent in Copenhagen.[38] While fecal transit time was similar in both locations, stool bulk was higher in Kuopio.

A review of seven highly regarded studies published in the 1980s, however, revealed inconsistent results for fiber.[39] At least one study, which showed a relation between fiber and frequency of colon cancer, suggested that only one of the many forms of fiber listed was associated with the disease. Recent research has suggested that low dietary fiber may also cause stomach, breast, ovarian, and endometrial cancers.[40] But studies attempting to correlate fiber intake with cancers other than colon have been few.

Other Dietary Items. Food additives, fats, the beta-carotene complex, and fiber are the best-known subjects in the area of diet and cancer. A complete list of food items known or thought to cause cancer would be long indeed. A few less familiar items balance those already discussed.

If "everybody knows" that hazardous chemicals, radiation, and low dietary fiber cause cancer, very few realize that "natural" foods consumed by Americans every day may contain even more potent carcinogens. These foods contain cancer-causing chemicals not added by farmers, processors, or distributors, but produced naturally by the plants themselves. In millions of years of evolution, many plants have acquired the ability to produce chemicals that act as natural pesticides. These agents protect against fungi, insects, and animal predators. One authority has remarked that "we are ingesting in our daily diet at least 10,000 times more natural pesticides than man-made pesticide residues."[41] Although only a few of these naturally occurring substances have been tested, it appears likely that many are carcinogens.

Several very familiar foods contain naturally occurring carcinogens.

Basil contains estragole, mushrooms contain hydrazines, brown mustard contains allyl isothiocyanate—all capable of causing cancer in laboratory animals. Celery contains psoralens, light-activated carcinogens that become more concentrated in the presence of mold. Molds, which frequently contaminate food substances, produce antibiotic materials to protect themselves from other microorganisms. These materials are frequently carcinogenic. Aflatoxin, an extremely powerful carcinogen produced by mold, is found in wheat, corn, nuts, peanuts, and other stored grains and seeds.[42]

Traditional methods of cooking and storing food may also raise cancer risks. Broiling and frying meat and fish can produce chemicals in the same class (polycyclic hydrocarbons) as those associated with cancer among the chimney sweeps of old and among today's roofers, gas workers, and coke-oven operatives. Consumption of fried, salted, or smoked fish or pickled vegetables appears to cause stomach cancer, perhaps because of the large amounts of salt these foods contain.[43] As the proportion of such items in the American diet has declined (and the consumption of fresh fruits and vegetables has increased), the frequency of stomach cancer has plummeted. Japanese-Americans in Hawaii—who, it would appear, consume an "Americanized" diet—have a much lower rate of stomach cancer than Japanese people living in Japan. The Japanese-Americans are genetically similar, but they consume a much lower proportion of smoked, pickled, and salted foods.

Finally, it is interesting to review the reported relationship between coffee drinking and cancer. A 1981 article in the prestigious *New England Journal of Medicine* compared Boston patients hospitalized for pancreatic cancer with those hospitalized for other reasons. To the consternation of coffee drinkers, patient interviews indicated that those who had pancreatic cancer habitually consumed more coffee than the comparison group.[44] But by 1986, the researchers had changed their minds, reporting in a larger study that coffee drinking was unrelated to cancer.[45]

LIFESTYLE AND BEHAVIOR

Important causes of cancer and opportunities for avoiding the disease seem to lie in the area of lifestyle and behavior. Even under the most constrained circumstances, Americans typically exercise substantial choice over their day-to-day activities and personal practices. Researchers have carried out numerous studies of the relationship between personal behavior and development of cancer. The areas of greatest importance include sexual practices, alcohol consumption, exercise, childbearing, and use of tobacco.

Sex. Certain sexual practices predispose women to developing cancer of the uterine cervix. These practices include early marriage, first pregnancy at a young age, sexual activity in early adolescence, and multiple sexual partners. Women who have histories of venereal disease face higher risks of cervical cancer. The disease tends to occur most frequently among minorities and economically disadvantaged people.

It is tempting to ask whether men face a similar risk of cancer as a result of promiscuous sex. Like cervical cancer, prostate cancer has been found more frequently among men who begin to have intercourse at an early age, have had many sexual partners, and have histories of venereal disease. Findings from a comparison of Catholic priests with other men in the Los Angeles area, however, contradict this hypothesis. Among five hundred deceased priests, thirteen were found to have died of prostate cancer. In a comparable population of male decedents, only eight such deaths would have been expected. The absence of a lower death rate from prostate cancer among men who were presumably celibate contradicts the belief that the disease is sexually transmitted.[46]

Childbearing. If promiscuous sex exposes women to greater cancer risks, having children may protect them. Pregnancy and childbirth seem to play a significant role in preventing cancers of the endometrium, ovary, and breast.[47] Generally, women who have full-term pregnancies experience fewer full ovulation cycles over the course of their lives than those who neither become pregnant nor have children. Reduction in the number of cycles, it appears, results in lower overall production of female gonad-stimulating hormones, which promote the growth of malignant tissues. The relation between hormone production and pregnancy is complex, however. Women who have never had children may have a lower cancer risk than those who first become mothers in their late thirties.

Exercise. People who exercise regularly may help protect themselves from some forms of cancer, particularly malignancies of the colon and breast. Several researchers have reported that sedentary people have greater risks of colon cancer than those who exercise regularly. Explanations have focused on the fact that exercise tends to stimulate peristalsis, which may in turn reduce contact time between carcinogens and the tissues that line the colon. Two studies by researchers at the University of Southern California compared sedentary and physically active individuals. One study compared men whose occupations required strenuous physical work with those in sedentary occupations. Men with sedentary jobs had an 80 percent greater risk of colon cancer than those with physically demanding jobs. A second study compared retirement community residents who reported exercising less than one hour per day with those averaging two or more hours per day. Among men, those with low activity developed colon cancer 2.3 times more often than the highly active; no difference was detected among women.[48]

Physical activity among women, particularly in girlhood or adolescence, has shown signs of helping protect against breast cancer. As with ovarian cancer, reduced hormone production may serve as the preventive mechanism. As noted earlier, a greater number of complete ovulation cycles (due to lack of interruption from pregnancy or to early commencement of the cycles) seems to coincide with a higher risk of certain cancers. Exercise in adolescence seems to delay the establishment of regular ovulation, reducing exposure to these hormones.[49]

Alcohol. A growing number of researchers have begun to suspect a connection between alcohol consumption and cancer. Physicians have known for some time that heavy drinkers develop cancers of the mouth, larynx, and esophagus more often than light drinkers or nondrinkers. But a series of studies in the 1980s suggests that light or social drinkers may also face an increased risk of breast cancer.[50] Although a definite link between light drinking and cancer has not been established, this possible risk is a continuing concern of researchers.

Tobacco. The fact that tobacco causes lung cancer is almost universally acknowledged. Tobacco receives attention here only to illustrate the magnitude of risk its use involves. Because the relationship between tobacco and cancer is so strong, and because its use is so widespread, it far and away represents the greatest overall cancer hazard discussed in this chapter. Authoritative studies indicate that about one-third of all cancer deaths in the United States around 1980 were caused by tobacco. A person who smokes twenty cigarettes per day beginning at age twenty has ten times the risk of developing lung cancer as a nonsmoker.[51] Tobacco use raises the chance not only of lung cancer but also of bladder, pancreatic, oral, laryngeal, pharyngeal, and esophogeal cancers. Use of tobacco multiplies the carcinogenic effect of other agents, sometimes greatly. The risk for cancer of the esophagus associated with moderate use of alcohol, for example, is three times greater among heavy smokers than among nonsmokers.[52] Risk increases of even greater magnitude have been observed for industrial carcinogens. Workers who both smoke and are exposed to asbestos or uranium-mine dusts, for example, experience astronomical lung cancer rates.

This already extensive list could continue indefinitely. Researchers on the exogenous causes of cancer have identified factors as exotic as parasites in undercooked snake meat consumed in Africa and Asia. They have reported phenomena as familiar to the public as the "epidemic" of cervical cancer in young women whose mothers received prescriptions of diethylstilbestrol (DES) during their pregnancies. Whether exotic or mundane, exogenous causes of cancer are of special interest because they are presumably avoidable.

Endogenous Causes of Cancer

The fact that many exogenous cancer risks can be avoided does not necessarily mean that cancer is an avoidable disease. Cancers are also caused by *endogenous* factors—those that arise within the body, often at the cellular or molecular level. These factors are typically less open to direct observation, manipulation, and avoidance than exogenous factors. A description of only a few of these factors illustrates their importance, independent of "environmental" influences.

AGE

Aging is at the same time the least avoidable part of life and the greatest cancer risk factor. Except for the few malignant diseases that occur exclusively among children, older people are more likely to develop cancer than younger ones. Age-group comparisons of Americans diagnosed with cancer between 1978 and 1981 illustrate this basic fact. Among those aged thirty through thirty-four years, the rate was 71 per 100,000; among those aged fifty through fifty-four, the rate was 501 per 100,000; among those seventy through seventy-four, it was 1,772 per 100,000. The climb was particularly steep for some forms of cancer. In colon cancer, for example, those aged fifty through fifty-four were diagnosed at the rate of 36 per 100,000, and those aged seventy through seventy-four were diagnosed at 216 per 100,000—an increase of 500 percent over twenty years. For prostate cancer, the rates were 12 per 100,000 and 247 per 100,000—an increase of 2,000 percent over twenty years. The trends for cancers of the cervix and larynx were less steep, increasing at 50 and 100 percent between these two age groups. But the trend is still sharply up. For leukemia, often considered a cancer of the young, the rate for people between thirty and thirty-four was 2.5 per 100,000; for those fifty through fifty-four, 9.8 per 100,000; for those seventy through seventy-four, 46.2 per 100,000.[53]

ENDOGENOUS HORMONES

Researchers have found evidence that endogenous hormones, those originating through spontaneous processes entirely within the body, contribute to the development of cancer. These investigators suspect that people who have excess concentrations of such hormones in the bloodstream are especially likely to contract certain cancers. Diseases known or believed to be linked to hormones include cancers of the endometrium, breast, prostate, ovary, testes, thyroid, and bone.

Scientists explain the relationship between hormones and cancer by suggesting that the same biological process that promotes normal growth also increases the risk of cancer. Hormones such as testosterone and estrogen promote the growth of tissues in specific "target" organs, such as the prostate and the breast. All tissues grow through the process of cell division. Every time a cell divides, "copying errors" in this DNA-guided process may produce a cancer cell. An excess of hormones accelerates growth, with each extra cell division raising the chance that a cancer cell will be produced.[54]

Of course, production of hormones associated with some forms of cancer seems to be promoted by exogenous factors as well, such as dietary fat intake (discussed in the preceding section). But processes entirely within the body, in the absence of any outside factor, can result in excess production of the hormones in question. These processes include the complex, coordinated actions of the brain, hypothalamus, and pituitary glands, which initiate and regulate production of the suspect hormones. Indeed, studies have shown that women known to be at risk for breast cancer have elevated levels of estrogen[55] and that men with prostatic cancer have elevated levels of testosterone.[56]

GENETICS AND HEREDITY

The influence of genetic heritage appears strong in many, perhaps most, forms of cancer. Both indirect and direct evidence supports the belief that heredity plays an important role in cancer. Physicians and scientists have known for many years that patients whose family members have had cancer are more likely to develop cancer themselves, although perhaps a different form of the disease. At the end of the twentieth century, moreover, scientists began to identify the actual biochemical mechanisms that predisposed the children of people who developed cancer to eventually contract the disease themselves.

Direct monitoring of patients and their families indicates a hereditary factor in colon, breast, and ovarian cancers, to cite only a few familiar instances. People with a near relative who has had colon cancer are three times as likely to develop it themselves as are people without such a relative.[57] Women whose mothers had breast cancer have three times the risk of contracting this illness as those whose mothers did not have the disease.[58] Women with mothers or sisters who have had breast, uterine, or ovarian cancer have five times the likelihood of contracting ovarian cancer as women without this family history.[59]

In the late twentieth century, the genes that cause cancer to be inherited were first isolated. Scientists initially identified a single gene that functions as a mechanism in development of retinoblastoma, a form of cancer capable of causing blindness. Damaged or deficient forms of this gene, which can be passed from generation to generation, actually cause the disease.[60] A massive project begun in the late twentieth century aimed at mapping the entire human genome, the 50,000 to 100,000 genes found in human cells, many more of which would surely be found to cause specific forms of cancer.

Still, the part played by heredity in cancer development is complex. Even at a single anatomical site, heredity seems to account for only some of the disease. It is not in the least unusual for people with no family history of breast cancer, colon cancer, retinoblastoma, or any other genetically linked cancer to develop these diseases.

Genetic factors appear capable of acting independently or in cooperation with exogenous ones as causes of cancer. A series of discoveries in 1990 illustrates this fact in relation to lung cancer.[61] Scientists identified a gene that, when activated, caused the body to transform chemicals found in cigarette smoke into powerful cancer-causing agents. People who inherited this gene were especially likely to develop lung cancer if they smoked. Smokers without this gene faced a lower risk, but still considerably higher than the risk faced by nonsmokers. At the same time, nonsmokers with the gene appeared more likely to develop lung cancer than nonsmokers without it.[62]

RACE

Finally, race has an important impact on risk of cancer. When all forms of cancer are considered together and the influence of age is controlled, blacks face a 10 percent higher risk than whites. The risks experienced by Japanese, Chinese, and Filipinos are 25 to 34 percent lower than the risks faced by whites. Interracial differences are greater for individual forms of cancer. Among men, blacks develop lung cancer 50 percent more often than whites, and prostate cancer 60 percent more often. White women develop breast cancer 20 percent more often than black women, but cancer of the cervix less than half as often.[63]

Researchers have attributed some but not all of these differences to social and economic differences between whites and blacks. In the 1980s, Americans with lower levels of income and education were especially likely to use tobacco. Black people, more often in the less advantaged income and education categories, were significantly more likely to smoke. Income and education "explained" part of the difference in cervical cancer. But after the influence of these socioeconomic factors had been taken into account, black women still experienced an elevated risk of the disease.[64]

This chapter describes endogenous causes of cancer in less detail than exogenous causes. Less discussion is needed. While many of the specific mechanisms remain mysteries, substantiation of the importance of the endogenous factors discussed in this chapter is generally more consistent than for the exogenous causes. It seems likely, for example, that most readers of this book can verify the importance of age and heredity as correlates if not actual causes of cancer on the basis of personal experience. While socioeconomic (exogenous) factors partially explain the influence of race, the suspicion remains strong that race reflects genetic predisposition (endogenous) to at least some forms of cancer. The influence of endogenous hormones on the development of at least some cancers is virtually certain.

The Limits of Cancer Prevention

The assertion that most cancer can be prevented has stronger roots in belief and hope than in fact. Scientists have identified some definite cancer hazards in industrial chemicals and radiation. But the number of people with significant exposure to these hazards is small. Investigators have assembled a sizable body of research on nutrition and cancer. But findings have been weak and results inconsistent. A few exogenous causes of cancer represent opportunities for prevention. But many are virtually impossible to avoid. During most human life spans, endogenous factors probably predominate over exogenous risks. Early estimates that 75 to 80 percent of all cancers are environmentally determined and thus avoidable now seem unrealistically high.

Individuals, health professionals, and public officials should exploit every opportunity to guard against known cancer risks that are, in fact, significant and avoidable. Of the factors examined in this chapter, three represent important cancer risks and involve widespread public exposure: tobacco, sunlight, and asbestos (see Table 1, column A). Smoking is the leading known cause of cancer in the United States today and is clearly an avoidable risk. Excessive exposure to sunlight, though widely thought to be harmless and even healthful, causes thousands of preventable cancers, many of them fatal. Asbestos, though recognized as a cancer hazard and the object of extensive abatement efforts, is still widespread in the environment.

But other environmental factors are either weak carcinogens at their usual levels of concentration or affect only scattered individuals in the population (see Table 1, column B). No proven industrial carcinogen other than asbestos and no high-level radiation hazard other than solar ultraviolet affect large numbers of Americans. Arsenic and benzene are industrial chemicals seldom if ever found in consumer goods. Cancer hazards from chemicals naturally occurring in food plants represent much greater risks than pesticide residues or saccharin. Natural carcinogens in a single raw mushroom produce a cancer hazard over a hundred times greater than the average American's daily exposure to PCBs. The estragole in a dried basil leaf poses almost twice the cancer risk of the saccharin in a twelve-ounce can of diet cola.[65]

The public and some health professionals may have placed much too great an emphasis on the hazards of low-level radiation. With the exception of those likely in a major nuclear war (after which acute problems

Table 1 *Exogenous Causes of Cancer (Proven or Suspected)*

A. Major Preventable Causes	B. Minor Preventable Causes	C. Uncertain or Unlikely Causes
(These known cancer causes affect a large number of people and are strong carcinogens)	*(These known cancer causes affect a limited number of people or are weak carcinogens)*	*(Although cited as causes, these factors have not been clearly demonstrated as carcinogens in humans)*
Tobacco Sunlight Asbestos	Ionizing radiation (medical, experimental, industrial sources) Industrial chemicals Pesticide residues Heavy alcohol use Maternal diethylstilbestrol (DES) Early promiscuous sex (females only) Salted fish and meats High-fat diet Diet low in beta-carotene	Low-fiber diet Sedentary lifestyle Magnetic fields Saccharin Nitrites Coffee

would eclipse cancer as a health concern), cancer risks associated with man-made radiation seem to be minor. Commenting on the results of his team's research on cancer in the parts of Utah affected by fallout from bomb tests in the 1950s and early 1960s, Dr. Walter Stevens noted that "any large-scale effect should be apparent by now. . . . In fact, I don't see a major hazard. I don't see anything I would be overly worried about."[66]

With respect to the population as a whole, the greatest hazards from ionizing radiation seem to come from (1) medical and dental X rays and (2) natural sources—namely, background radiation from solid radioactive elements and their compounds, radon gas, and cosmic rays. Most people will undoubtedly continue to undergo X-ray examinations. Better ventilation and basement construction may abate radon exposure in the home. But other natural sources of radiation are probably unavoidable.

Research on dietary cancer risks may eventually prove important for some specific diseases. Beta-carotene may well help prevent lung cancer, and a low-fat diet may reduce the risk of colon cancer. But studies of the relationships between fat and breast cancer, and between fiber and colon cancer, have failed to demonstrate definite benefits. Generally, research findings available in the late twentieth century offered little in the way of incontrovertible guidance for direct action.

Research on hormones and cancer implies an important role for behavior and lifestyle. The image of girls' exercising regularly in adolescence, having a limited number of children in early adulthood, and adhering to a low-fat diet as the years pass is appealingly wholesome. But whether many will establish and maintain this lifestyle for the purpose of avoiding breast and reproductive malignancies is in doubt. In any case, entirely unrelated processes within the body may affect hormone secretion and metabolism, and the ultimate likelihood of cancer, to a much greater degree.

Whatever the impact of environmental chemicals, radiation, diet, or lifestyle, basic biological processes occurring at the cellular or molecular level seem to play an important and independent role. As Dr. Charles McKann has commented, "the process by which cells normally divide and reproduce themselves is extremely complicated and mistakes can occur without any outside inducement whatsoever, and these mistakes can evolve into cancer. I think this is probably the source of a large number of *spontaneous* cancers in humans." And further, "It is quite possible that environmental factors contribute to the cause of 15 to 20 percent of all cancers, but not 80 percent. Most cancers probably arise spontaneously, with no significant outside cause." McKann dismisses the 80 percent estimate as "very wild talk."[67]

Scientists today can only guess at the actual proportion of cancers that may be avoidable. Comparison of some known rates of occurrence due to behavioral and hereditary factors provides a perspective. One study has indicated that lack of exercise increases risk of colon cancer among men by a factor of 2.3; with the addition of the women studied (among whom there was no effect), the risk increased by a factor of less than twofold.[68] This finding compares with a threefold increase in risk of colon cancer for family members of people with the disease.[69] Even in lung cancer, where the strongest of exogenous factors (smoking) is crucial, endogenous factors play an important role. At age fifty, a nonsmoker who carries the gene now suspected of causing predisposition to lung cancer has a risk of developing the disease about eight times greater than a nonsmoker who does not carry the gene. This increase in risk is about the same as that of a fifty-year-old who smokes but does not carry the gene.[70]

In all, less than 50 percent of the cancer cases that occurred in the United States around the close of the twentieth century seem to have arisen from exogenous causes. Aging, heredity, and accidents in cell reproduction are powerful factors in the development of cancer. Some cancers linked with environmental causes, moreover, are still not preventable; many environmental hazards, such as nitrites and cosmic rays, are virtually unavoidable.

Even the most familiar and compelling of scientific findings on prevention seem to involve controversy when applied in the real world. The properties of spinach are illustrative. Spinach is rich in presumably beneficial beta-carotene. But the vegetable also contains high levels of nitrites, believed to promote formation of carcinogens in the body. Scientists in the late twentieth century were experimenting with the drug tamoxifen to prevent breast cancer. Because it blocked the action of estrogen and simulated the effects of pregnancy, tamoxifen appeared capable of reducing the incidence of the disease. But scientists also warned that tamoxifen could promote bone loss and raise the risk of heart disease in otherwise healthy women.[71] Critics have even questioned the honored place of asbestos in the hierarchy of carcinogens, contending that only one of the forms in which the mineral occurs is truly hazardous.[72]

Behavioral and environmental explanations of cancer have captured the American public's imagination. The idea of prevention falls on fertile cultural soil in the United States, whose values emphasize individual initiative and responsibility for one's own well-being. The popularity of such thinking is strengthened by the emphasis placed on physical attractiveness, fitness, and youth. It has resulted in widespread beliefs about exogenous causes of cancer that have found little consistent support in scientific research (see Table 1, column C). The most important answers to the question "Who survives cancer?" must be sought in other areas.

Postscript on Prevention:
Heart Disease and Cancer

A comparison of cancer with heart disease highlights what may be an essential difficulty in reducing mortality through prevention—namely, that cancer rates may, in the long run, prove more stubbornly resistant to large-scale prevention efforts than those of other serious illnesses.

In the mid-twentieth century, scientists identified several of the same factors as important in prevention of both cancer and heart disease. These included tobacco, fatty foods, and sedentary lifestyle. Alert to these scientific findings, many Americans quit smoking, reduced fats in their diet, and began to exercise regularly. Rates of death from heart attacks and associated conditions fell steadily—declining by about one-fifth between 1968 and 1978, for example, among Americans aged thirty to seventy-four years.[73] Researchers have uncovered strong evidence that this decline occurred largely because people had fewer heart attacks, not because they received more effective medical care after the attacks.[74] Many physicians and public health officials are convinced that avoidance of tobacco, dietary fat, and sedentary habits accounts for the drop in occurrence of heart attacks and deaths associated with them.

But at the same time, both sickness and death from cancer became more common. From 1973 to 1981, the rate of cancer cases diagnosed among Americans rose by 13 percent; even when the increasing age of the population was taken into account, the rate increased by 8.5 percent in this short period. Between 1962 and 1982, the rate of cancer deaths among Americans increased by 25 percent; when the influence of the aging trend was controlled, the death rate still increased by 8.7 percent.[75] If the trend toward a healthier way of life in the United States had begun to reduce the risk of heart attacks, it had made no impact on the increasing cancer threat.

This observation raises the possibility that the death rate from cancer may ultimately prove more resistant to preventive efforts than the rate from heart disease. A recent report on smoking, heart disease, and lung cancer adds evidence in this direction. This report was based on the well-known study called MRFIT (Multiple Risk Factor Intervention Trial), which followed 12,866 men for over ten years to assess the effects of habits and lifestyle on longevity. Men who were smokers when they entered the study faced elevated risk of both heart attacks and lung cancer. During the course of the study, many of the smokers successfully quit. Those who quit experienced an immediate drop in their risk of dying from a heart attack but, for several years, continued to face the same high risk of death from lung cancer as those who persisted in smoking.[76] In at least one common risk factor, avoidance of the hazard brings much more immediate benefits for heart attack than for cancer survival.

♦   ♦   ♦   ♦   ♦

It is undeniable that many cancers can be prevented. But efforts to reduce cancer mortality should not aim primarily at prevention. Everyone concerned with cancer as a threat to survival must pay close attention to exogenous causes and environmental risks. Still, even the best-informed and most conscientious individual faces a significant risk of cancer. Like cancer treatment, cancer prevention is ineffective in many areas and is likely to remain so well into the twenty-first century. Even the best-planned and best-executed cancer prevention campaign will probably never achieve a reduction of cancer mortality approaching 50 percent. Potential preventability of cancer should not eclipse the importance of treatment.

In the twentieth century, the biological sciences added significantly to humankind's knowledge of cancer. Effective treatment became available for many forms of the disease. Physicians could significantly extend the lives of many people for whom no "cure" was available. Scientists identified a wide variety of factors that made some people more likely to develop cancer than others. But, as Chapters 3 and 4 of this book suggest, physicians and biomedical scientists have not defined a clear path to further major improvements in cancer survival. Breakthroughs of practical and immediate significance in cancer treatment do not seem ready to spring from the research laboratories. Most causes of cancer do not seem readily removable from the human organism or its environment.

In the light of these limitations, activities outside the concerns of traditional science grow in importance. Major improvements in cancer survival seem likely only as a consequence of developments in thinking, behavior, and conditions of life. Today's potential and actual cancer patients can improve their chances of survival by obtaining appropriate medical care. But it seems likely that a wide range of personal decisions, behavior patterns, and outside constraints prevent many from doing so in a timely manner. In addition, a growing circle of influential practitioners and commentators contend that a shift of emphasis in health care from technical intervention to psychological amelioration will improve survival in many serious illnesses, including (and perhaps especially) cancer.

Chapters 5 through 8 examine a series of factors which, though largely outside the perspective of traditional biomedical science, are potentially crucial in determining who survives cancer. The following chapter addresses the most basic of these: the mood and outlook of cancer patients.

CHAPTER FIVE

Emotional Health and Cancer Survival

No one can ignore the possibility that emotional factors may affect survival among the ill. Philosophers and theologians through the ages have counseled against distinguishing too sharply between mind and body. The question of whether emotions affect cancer survival lies outside the usual concerns of modern biology and medicine. But the realization that neither technical breakthroughs nor preventive measures will soon eliminate cancer as a major cause of mortality underscores the importance of new alternatives. The remainder of this book will concentrate on factors that involve thinking, behavior, and conditions of life. Despite the achievements of biomedical science in cancer, these factors may, for many individuals in the century to come, make the real difference between life and death.

Scientists encounter major difficulties when they attempt to assess the impacts of emotions, behavior, and social and economic conditions on cancer survival. Psychologists, sociologists, and economists work with information that is considerably "softer" than that of the more traditional sciences. Engineers have developed instruments capable of very accurately assessing clinical facts such as the concentration of blood gases and enzymes. But social scientists must usually ask people questions in order to obtain data on their personal habits, states of mind, family incomes, and cultural beliefs. The uniqueness of each human being makes it hazardous to compare one person's response with that of another. Individual human beings interpret questions differently and, in their answers, may express the same thought in different words. Unlike a laboratory autoanalyzer, moreover, a human subject responding to a questionnaire may at any time elect to lie.

Health professionals and social commentators with interests in the relationship between emotions and cancer have labored against these difficulties. Many have bypassed the cautious methods upon which scientists have traditionally insisted. Collections of anecdotes have been widely used in attempts to demonstrate connections between cancer survival and personality, outlook, and mood. Otherwise, proponents of the emotional theory have looked to the traditional sciences, citing principles and studies that appear to support their belief in a link between emotions and survival. Some scientific studies have focused directly on the relationships of emotional factors to cancer survival. But only a few have been carried out under rules of observation, measurement, and analysis comparable in rigor to those of clinical trials. People who believe in a relationship between psychological factors and cancer survival have never based their position primarily on such studies.

The Seattle Longitudinal Assessment of Cancer Survival (SLACS) serves as an important resource in improving understanding of the role that emotions—as well as other aspects of thinking, behavior, and conditions of life—may actually play in determining who survives cancer. As detailed in Appendix A, the SLACS is a long-term study of survival of people diagnosed with one of four common cancers: malignancies of the lung, pancreas, prostate, and uterine cervix. The SLACS followed 536 people, a large number in comparison with most studies of psychosocial aspects of cancer. The study obtained vast amounts of data on the lives, resources, and problems of these individuals, most elicited through extensively validated, quantitative scales, designed to minimize subjectivity. The SLACS included a battery of detailed questions to detect psychological distress. The resulting accumulation of information has provided an opportunity to study the relationship of psychosocial factors—particularly the emotional states of patients—to cancer survival more comprehensively and rigorously than ever before.

Documentation of a strong relationship between emotional factors and cancer survival would have important implications for treatment. Just as some believe that preventive efforts should replace the current emphasis on finding a cancer cure, others contend that spiritual and psychological interventions may be more effective than traditional medicine at curing cancer. In view of their powerful implications, emotional theories of cancer survival require objective assessment.

Two types of inquiry provide a basis for assessing the strength of the theory linking emotions and cancer survival. The first is a review of the cultural underpinnings of the theory. Rather than science, deep-seated beliefs among American and some European thinkers have given rise to this popular approach to explaining cancer mortality. The second is a close examination of actual scientific studies of emotional factors and survival, with special attention to the studies that most closely approximate the rigor of traditional clinical trials.

The Emotional Theory of Survival

Many popular writers today tell their audiences that psychological factors predispose people to contracting cancer and that improved emotional health enables cancer patients to recover. The field of behavioral medicine, which looks to psychological techniques for solutions to organic health problems, is in the forefront of this thinking. Michael A. Lerner, a leading exponent of this perspective, makes a firm connection between the cancer patient's emotions and his or her chances for recovery. Discussing the benefits of group therapy sessions for cancer patients, he writes: "You become different from the person who developed the cancer. Becoming different personally may change the environment the cancer grew in; it may become so inhospitable that the cancer shrinks."[1]

This kind of thinking finds considerable sympathy in the American public. Every family, in fact, seems to have its own anecdote. A grandfather, mother, sibling was diagnosed with cancer. Doctors called the condition hopeless and sadly informed the family that the patient had less than a year to live. But the relative outlived the doctors' predictions, by six months, a whole year, several years. The survivor had an extraordinary "will to live," the family often explains. The doctors could not appreciate this "fighting spirit." A kind of mystical gift helped the individual triumph over dread disease. Indeed, the family might add, this spirit, outlook, or gift appeared in many aspects of the person's life and relations with others. The relative's ability to "beat" cancer was just one more manifestation of his or her basic personal capabilities, talents, and blessings.

Professional and popular support for a psychological explanation of cancer survival reflects the strong tradition of individualism in America. Generally, Americans seek the causes of individual success and misfortune within the individual. The tradition of individualism extends to the worlds of academic achievement, work, family stability—and, increasingly, to health. The millions of joggers, dieters, and voluntary psychiatric clients in America today attest to this tradition's persistence. The appeal of prevention as an approach to cancer owes at least part of its strength to this individualism. Like fitness and self-care, prevention offers people a means of avoiding the disease by taking action on their own behalf.

Few if any would dispute the importance of individual attitudes toward disease, feelings about oneself, or willingness to take steps to ameliorate or overcome personal misfortune. Few, moreover, would exclude from the realm of legitimate medicine techniques designed to reduce the cancer patient's level of anxiety or depression. A good family physician should pay sufficient attention to both the observable lesion and the patient's perceived comfort. But those seeking to understand the factors that increase or reduce cancer survival must question psychologically based theories, despite their appeal to basic American values. It is essential to examine the cultural heritage on which this approach is based, and the scientific studies to which its proponents have looked for support.

Culture and the Psychology of Survival

Speculation about relationships between the mind and cancer predates modern medicine and extends beyond the ranks of American individualists and orthodox medical practitioners. A number of classical medical sages, including Galen, believed that sadness, depression, and "melancholia" led to cancer. Women were thought to be especially susceptible to contracting cancer for emotional reasons. While these sages contributed much to the development of modern medicine, it is also important to remember that they had no knowledge of germ theory or biochemistry and treated their patients with mineral baths and bloodletting.

In modern times, German psychologist Wilhelm Reich did much to publicize the notion that psychological factors cause cancer, linking the disease with sexual repression. Although intermittently popular in the United States, Reich was eventually jailed for fraudulent promotion of a device to enhance sexual capacity. Reich died, discredited and destitute, in a mental hospital. His influence has periodically resurfaced, however, and his name appears now and then in popular psychology.

Practitioners in better standing than Reich have helped disseminate the notion that mental condition can contribute to the risk of cancer or affect the cancer patient's chances for survival. In the 1970s, a series of works by physicians and psychologists linked cancer incidence and survival with lassitude and isolation during childhood,[2] self-pity and an inability to retain close relationships,[3] and apathy, self-contempt, and the feeling that life holds no more hope.[4]

But the principal source of popular belief in a relationship between state of mind and cancer has almost certainly been culture rather than science. In the late 1970s, critic and essayist Susan Sontag reviewed a broad range of cultural elements that link emotions with physical disease.[5] At the most basic level, these elements include the language of everyday discussion in which people describe and conceptualize illness. They also occur in "high culture," as themes running through novels and poetry that associate depression, pessimism, and a negative outlook on life with fatal disease.

Sontag's essay focuses primarily on two diseases, tuberculosis and cancer. Culture has tended to transform both diseases, tuberculosis in the nineteenth century and cancer in the twentieth, from objective clinical entities into emotionally charged cultural themes. In their respective eras, science could not adequately explain these diseases and medicine could not cure them. They came to be perceived as insidious, mysterious, and hopeless. These supposed qualities made them attractive to commentators and writers as metaphors for describing people and social phenomena. Persons who contracted these diseases were, in turn, believed to possess the secretive and hopeless qualities that the diseases represented in literature.

Writers of the nineteenth and early twentieth centuries associated peculiarly positive qualities with the secretiveness and hopelessness attributed to tuberculosis. The literary genre took tuberculosis to be an expression of frustrated passion. Writers in this tradition most often traced such frustration to unfulfilled love. Keats, for example, attributed his "consumption" to separation from his mistress. Tuberculosis could be caused not only by thwarted love but also—particularly among the creatively inspired—by poverty. Mimi in *La Bohème* exemplifies this etiology. Both varieties of frustration appeared to involve self-renunciation by the high-minded. In this respect, tuberculosis was perceived as a "noble" form of illness. The nineteenth-century metaphor presented tuberculosis, a disease identified with the chest and upper body, as an affliction of the soul.

Tuberculosis, according to Sontag, lost its appeal as a literary fantasy with the development of definitive treatment in the twentieth century, and was replaced by cancer as a metaphor in language and literature. Metaphorically, cancer shares the secretiveness, insidiousness, and hopelessness once attributed to tuberculosis. In this metaphor, cancer is also associated with spiritual deprivation. But instead of a noble frustration of acknowledged passion, cancer is viewed as stemming from denial of passion, suppression of anger, stifling of creativity, repression (into the Freudian "unconscious") of desire, and personal defeat. In contemporary discourse, one hears of cancer as an "invasion," people who contract cancer as "victims," efforts to develop cures as "crusades." Political discussion has adopted cancer as a metaphor to describe evil imposed from without. It is a small logical step to explaining the individual's developing or succumbing to cancer as an absence of "life force," an unwillingness or spiritual inability to fight the invader.

Sontag's analysis suggests that the mysteries, fantasies, and personal attributes encompassed by the cancer metaphor make no more sense than the obsolete metaphor surrounding tuberculosis. She writes: "As once TB was thought to come from too much passion, afflicting the reckless and sensual, today many people believe that cancer is a disease of insufficient passion, afflicting those who are sexually repressed, inhibited, unspontaneous, incapable of expressing anger. These seemingly opposite diagnoses are actually not so different versions of the same view (and deserve, in my opinion, the same amount of credence)."[6]

Sontag implies that the need for disease metaphors to express our fears about personal insufficiency, social change, and political instability will outlast the serviceability of cancer for that purpose. In the meantime, she suggests, the belief that personality flaws cause cancer or reduce survival chances amounts to a distasteful exercise in "blaming the victim."

What Sontag views as a mere fantasy destined to be abandoned with the development of improved cancer treatment, however, has achieved perhaps unprecedented popularity through the work of a literary figure of comparable stature. Norman Cousins's recollection of his personal experience with illness became a best-selling critique of medicine in the 1980s.[7] Cousins was hospitalized for a progressive, debilitating illness that his physicians were unable to diagnose. He soon became frustrated with his care and surroundings, turned to literature recommending "the full exercise of the affirmative emotions as a factor in enhancing body chemistry," and accordingly changed his environment and treatment regimen. In a now well-known search for recovery, Cousins left the hospital and moved to a nearby hotel. The move both improved the comfort of his surroundings and reduced the cost of his care. But most important, Cousins claims to have developed a program to trigger "affirmative emotions" through laughter, with the aid of comic literature and Groucho Marx films. Cousins apparently recovered, concluding that "the will to live is not a theoretical abstraction but a physiologic reality with therapeutic characteristics."[8]

Cousins himself did not agree with the conclusion that he "laughed" his way out of a crippling disease that doctors thought was irreversible. But his report is widely interpreted in that way. Several "experimental" programs, in fact, have been initiated to apply the principles "established" by Cousins's experience, most often focusing on patients hospitalized with advanced malignancies.

A prolific writer and longtime editor of the *Saturday Review of Literature*, Cousins had cultural rather than scientific credentials. He based his comments largely on personal experience—reporting, for example, a newfound ability to sleep after viewing a Groucho Marx movie. Although he cited scientific studies, he did not claim to be scientific and did not make specific recommendations for treatment. In the late twentieth century, however, clinicians began to offer emotionally based treatment regimens on the basis of evidence no more substantial than that cited in Cousins's writings.

Psychotherapy for Cancer

Cousins's description of his illness points out serious shortcomings in modern medical care. He had no scientific proof that he actually "cured himself with laughter." But he raised important issues about the priorities of medicine in the late twentieth century. The technical capabilities of medicine in this era often far outran concerns for the patient's comfort and dignity.

Influential writers and practitioners have developed methods of therapy consistent with this thinking. Dr. O. Carl Simonton is the most famous of these practitioners. Simonton states his view of the importance of emotions in cancer as follows:

It is our central premise that an illness is not purely a physical problem but rather a problem of the whole person, that it includes not only body but mind and emotions. We believe that emotional and mental states play a significant role both in *susceptibility* to disease, including cancer, and in *recovery* from all disease. We believe that cancer is often an indication of problems elsewhere in an individual's life, problems aggravated or compounded by a series of stresses six to eighteen months prior to the onset of cancer. The cancer patient has typically responded to these problems and stresses with a deep sense of hopelessness, or "giving up." This emotional response, we believe, in turn triggers a set of physiological responses that suppress the body's natural defenses and make it susceptible to producing abnormal cells.[9]

Simonton and his colleagues have applied this perspective in a well-known therapeutic program. At their Fort Worth Center, they conduct a program designed to stimulate the psychological processes believed to promote recovery from cancer. The program utilizes several "mental imagery techniques," which aim to strengthen patients' belief in their treatment, their body's natural defenses, and their ability to solve the problems they had before becoming ill. Simonton and his followers believe that creating alternative imaging will improve chances for recovery by increasing immune activity and decreasing abnormal cell production.

Individuals may carry out the six-week Simonton program on their own or through many hospitals. It begins with a prescription for reading books that explain the "interrelatedness of mind, body, and emotions." The program continues with exercises to overcome stress and resentment, promote commitment to recovery, explore feelings about death, and set goals for the future. Explicit imagery is apparently quite important. Among their successful patients, the Simonton team presents individuals who thought of their radiation treatments as volleys of bullets and their white blood corpuscles as sharks eating cancer cells.

Simonton and his colleagues use mostly anecdotal evidence to support the merits of their treatment method. They describe patients with the proper attitudes who experienced complete remissions from cancer or lived "many months beyond" their prognoses. They cite the familiar "placebo effect" as indirect support. They describe, for example, a man who received the experimental drug Krebiozen in the 1950s. The patient, they report, made steady progress until he learned that research studies had proven the drug ineffective. Only positive beliefs, they conclude, could have explained the patient's improvement followed by decline.

Simonton, Cousins, and other popular writers who explain cancer survival in terms of positive emotions do make reference to "research studies" in their books and speeches. Usually, though, these references are brief and lack detail about the conduct of the research or possible problems in its interpretation. People reading or listening for inspiration or entertainment may find these vague obeisances to the authority of science reassuring. But those who are seriously concerned with identifying who survives cancer and what may be done to increase an individual's chances must go considerably further.

Determining the real value of the emotional theory of cancer—and, just as important, its potential applicability in cancer therapy—requires detailed examination of scientific studies. Like lawyers arguing a case, commentators on health and medical care often select only those studies from the vast scientific literature that support the positions they favor. A practitioner with a particular point of view may convince an unwary reader on the basis of research reports that are fundamentally flawed. People who have a serious need to obtain accurate information on what genuinely *works* in cancer treatment must assess the strength of research cited to support a particular therapeutic approach, and weigh these studies against those that may support an opposing opinion.

What Do the Studies Really Say?

Proponents of the emotional theory of cancer survival have tended to draw selectively on studies done in the 1960s and 1970s by scientists in many fields. Some of these studies are well designed and executed, but others are scientifically very weak. Some of the investigations have focused directly on human survival; others, on organisms or life forms quite distant from human beings. Of the studies that appear generally acceptable to the scientific community, some seem to support the psychological theory of survival, others contradict the theory, and still others have proven inconclusive.

LABORATORY RESEARCH

Cousins, Simonton, and others of their persuasion regularly allude to laboratory research to support their assertions. This type of research engenders respect because it sounds like real science. It takes place in a setting presumably equipped with the traditional scientific trappings—glassware, chemical reagents, electronic measurement devices. Researchers perform experiments that expose tissues to factors thought to produce or inhibit cancer, and perform tests utilizing objective measurements and standard statistical techniques to see whether the stimuli had the expected results.

Laboratory scientists have, of course, performed many experiments to test theories that changes in body chemistry can cause or control cancer. Studies of this kind have concentrated, first, on the immune system. It is believed that a healthy immune system can identify and destroy cancer cells, which, like bacteria or viruses, are foreign bodies. Scientists have also focused their attention on hormones. Distributed through the bloodstream to tissues all over the body, these substances coordinate the actions of a variety of organs and affect cancer cells in important ways. As discussed in Chapters 3 and 4, established treatment methods include hormone manipulation for several cancers, and hormones are suspected as causes of some forms of the disease. Mainstream cancer research has focused strongly on the immune system in the search for new treatments.

Some experiments have addressed the possibility that emotions affect the immune system, and thus the ability of the body to fight cancer. This theory is especially important because some scientists think the body regularly produces a small number of cancer cells. If the immune system spots the abnormal cell and deals with it effectively, no tumor develops. Visible disease occurs only when the immune system breaks down. Advocates of this theory have reasoned that emotional stress causes cancer by interfering with the immune system.

An experiment by two laboratory investigators in the late 1960s illustrates the type of study often cited as evidence that emotions affect the immune system.[10] These investigators injected bovine serum albumin (BSA) into mice bred specifically for experimental purposes. It was known that each mouse's immune system would recognize this substance as foreign and would produce antibodies to destroy it. The experimenters wished to identify factors that affected the mouse immune system's response to the substance. One factor was the housing conditions under which the mice were kept. Some shared their cages with five other mice; others were kept alone.

After several weeks, the scientists tested blood samples from the mice for evidence of immune response. They reported that the mice kept in isolation had weaker immune responses than those kept in cages with other mice. They concluded that the psychological consequences of isolation accounted for the differences. These findings, they commented, "demonstrate for the first time that injection of a foreign protein in mice involves an immunological response that can be affected by the psycho-physiological experience accompanying separation from other mice."[11]

Hormones constitute the second major subject of laboratory-based research on relationships between emotions and cancer. The theory linking human feelings and behavior with cancer via the intervention of hormones is compelling. Everyone knows that anxiety, fear, and antic-ipation of certain stimuli cause changes in pulse rate, blood pressure, and glandular secretions. This is the basis for the polygraph lie detector, which records physiological changes in response to stress produced by untruthful testimony. Actual or anticipated misfortune or happiness apparently stimulates nervous reactions, which in turn activate the hypo-thalamus and pituitary glands. These kingpins in the body's biochemis-try cause several other glands to secrete hormones—most notably, ste-roids by the adrenals. In essence, this is a description of the familiar "fight-or-flight" response that all animals have to threats in their en-vironment.

Furthermore, scientists have demonstrated important connections between hormones and cancer. Some female cancers—such as endo-metrial and uterine malignancies—can develop only in the presence of stimulation by estrogen, a female sex hormone. Likewise, scientists have linked breast cancer with high concentrations of estrogens. In men, prostate cancers are dependent on the androgens, or male sex hormones. Prostate cancer never develops in their absence. Scientists have identified a wide variety of additional hormones—many of which are secreted in response to emotional stimulation—as growth factors in these and other cancers.[12]

But scientists investigating the relationship between emotions and resistance to disease have not always come to the same conclusions. Some research findings suggest that conditions associated with emo-tional disturbance may actually *increase* an animal's resistance to a wide range of illnesses, including cancer. While some researchers report that mice housed alone have a weaker immunological response than mice housed in groups, others find that solitary mice develop greater re-sistance to certain parasitic diseases than mice housed with other mice.[13] Some studies report that mice who fight with other mice have greater resistance to disease than tranquil members of their species. But other experiments indicate that fighting mice develop *decreased* resistance to illness. Likewise, basic science research on immune factors and hormones has major inconsistencies. The body's immune system fights disease, and an increase in its capabilities protects the individual from cancer—or so it would seem. But the authors of one study remark, "It is now believed that the development and course of only some tumors are restricted by immune activity and that immune factors may actually stimulate tumor growth under certain conditions."[14]

Increased hormone secretions—particularly those produced by the cortex areas of the adrenal glands—are associated with the growth of cancer. But research also documents beneficial effects from the presence of such hormones. Some of these agents are extensively used in cancer therapy. Patients whose tumor cells have molecular configurations capable of binding to these hormones have increased chances of responding positively to therapy.[15]

Clinicians who look to behavioral and emotional factors to help patients survive cancer try to back up their claims with laboratory experiments reported in the scientific journals. In fact, these experiments leave undecided the question of whether—and, perhaps even more important, how—emotions affect cancer. On the biochemical level, the relationships between cancer survival and immune factors and hormones are very complicated. Intense research in these areas continues. Impacts of immune factors and hormones differ from disease to disease. The final answer may never be known. Experiments focusing on emotional stimuli and behavior, moreover, do not give clear messages applicable to humans. How do crowded housing conditions and fighting behavior among mice translate into emotions experienced by people? Do humans fare better emotionally in cramped city apartments or roomy suburban homes? Should we consider isolation stressful, as it may be to shipwrecked sailors, or serenely pacifying, as it seems to religious hermits? Does fighting behavior stated in human terms signify anger and hostility or a healthful release of pent-up feelings?

Laboratory studies cannot answer the question of whether emotional well-being helps people survive cancer. In attempts to add stress to the environments of mice, monkeys, and other small mammals, biomedical experimenters have resorted to a variety of mechanisms, including crowding, food deprivation, and electric shocks. These conditions may change the animals' body chemistries. But to what, if any, *human* emotions do these animal reactions correspond? The chemical and nervous responses in animals may affect their resistance to bacteria or parasites to which the scientists expose them. But there are immense differences between these simple responses and the highly complex immunology of cancer. Studies in the laboratory have thus far failed to move the connection between emotional distress and cancer survival beyond anecdotes and theories. Real progress requires that scientists observe people with cancer, assess their emotional states, and monitor their survival.

HUMAN SURVIVAL STUDIES

Scientists have in fact done human studies, employing different techniques from the experiments just described. Unlike laboratory animals, people will seldom let experimenters subject them to noxious stimuli. Scientists do not usually expose human subjects to disease, and certainly not to cancer. Instead, studies of human beings almost always focus on patients already diagnosed with cancer. Researchers perform psychological tests on cancer patients and use the test results to predict the patient's survival time. Hospitals and specialized cancer treatment centers serve as research sites. Already having undergone much testing and many medical procedures, these patients often make willing (or at least compliant) study participants. Medical records that are regularly updated tell the investigators how long each patient lives after his or her diagnosis.

These studies almost always employ standardized tests developed by psychologists and psychiatrists to indicate emotional well-being or distress. The tests usually include series of questions asking the subject whether he or she feels hopeless, sad, blue, suspicious, withdrawn, happy, or satisfied. Other types of questions may request subjects to select preferences—"going out to see friends" versus "staying home and watching television," for example. They may ask the individual to describe some aspect of his or her behavior or social surroundings and resources. Responses to the questions are grouped into indices. Each index is designed to reflect a psychological characteristic, such as tension, depression, anger, resignation, or isolation. Psychiatrists have developed indices to measure syndromes such as neuroticism and paranoia. One large-scale test—known as the Minnesota Multiphasic Personality Inventory, or MMPI—has been given to countless college students, military recruits, and job applicants over several generations to assess fitness for special tasks and identify emotional problems.

It is difficult to believe that questions as simple as the ones appearing on these forms can measure complex human attributes. But they have several highly useful qualities. Because they are standardized, they allow for objective evaluation of individual moods and personalities. Being human themselves, clinicians may allow personal prejudices and "gut feeling" to influence their evaluations of certain patients. The indices themselves are validated by determining whether people with mood disturbance, neuroticism, etc., assessed according to alternative means, receive high scores on these indices.

The 1970s gave rise to a series of widely reported studies linking emotional characteristics with survival among cancer patients. A highly influential study assessed characteristics of women with breast cancer, including anxiety, hostility, depression, guilt, and "psychoticism."[16] A standard psychological test, the SCL-90-R, was used. The investigators reported that certain psychological characteristics were associated with long-term survival. But the report contained some major surprises. While Cousins, Simonton, and others in the behavioral medicine movement connected affirmative emotions with cancer survival, this study connected survival with what must be termed negative emotions. The report indicated that the long-term survivors had higher levels of anxiety, hostility, and psychoticism than the short-term survivors. They also had poorer attitudes and more hostility toward their physicians.

A study of patients with malignant melanoma, a highly aggressive form of skin cancer, produced similar results.[17] This study used a "melanoma adjustment scale" to predict relapse after surgery. On this scale, patients were asked to rate from 1 to 100 the amount of personal adjustment needed to cope with their life-threatening disease. If a great deal of personal adjustment had been required, the subject indicated a high number on the scale. The study found that the higher the score on the melanoma adjustment scale, the less likely the individual would be to experience a relapse. Again, fundamentally negative rather than positive emotions seem to correlate with a better prognosis in cancer. People who feel they are undergoing substantial personal adjustment appear likely to encounter more stress, depression, and disruption of lifestyle than those able to take their disease in stride.

The authors of both the breast cancer and the melanoma studies make an effort to interpret their results in a manner consistent with the tenets of behavioral medicine. According to the authors of the breast cancer study, the higher levels of anxiety and hostility really reflect a "fighting spirit," which may explain the tendency to survive. The authors of the melanoma study say that a higher "adjustment rating" may indicate greater willingness to acknowledge and confront the disease. In a rhetorical manipulation of major proportions, anxiety, hostility, and a difficult process of adjustment are thus transformed into positive emotions capable of increasing the patient's chances for survival. It seems far more likely, however, that these findings actually reflect neither firm nor especially meaningful research results. In both studies, the number of patients followed is extremely small (thirty-five in the breast cancer study and sixty-seven in the melanoma study), raising the possibility that the findings may be entirely accidental. Both studies followed patients for only one year. In all, neither the breast cancer nor the melanoma study collected enough data.

The breast cancer study has several other difficulties. The "long-term" survivors (those who survived for one year) were on the average six years younger than the ones who lived less than a year. Longer-term survival could have been traced simply to the age differences. All things being equal, younger people will always outlive their elders. Younger people, moreover, are more likely to criticize and make demands on their physicians. Finally, people who are healthier, and thus less likely to die soon, appear more likely to have the strength and motivation required to express tension and exhibit hostility—to their doctors or anyone else.

Few other studies remedy these shortcomings. An English researcher and his colleagues followed breast cancer patients for up to ten years.[18] His psychological tests led him to conclude that "optimistic attitudes" predicted survival. In his study, patients who looked upon their breast surgery as inconsequential or merely precautionary tended to survive longer. However, this study followed only fifty-seven patients. In addition, it leaves open the question that underlying disease may affect the patient's responses to the psychological tests. A breast cancer patient with more serious disease is less likely to interpret her illness or treatment as minor, and also is less likely to survive long-term.

The pronouncements of several distinguished and widely read authors exemplify a strong popular belief in America today—namely, that positive emotions increase an individual's chances of surviving cancer. Both literary figures and physicians subscribing to this belief often refer to research to support their contentions. The examples presented above typify the research these proponents cite in their writings. But none of the studies examined here provides convincing arguments that emotional well-being improves cancer survival. Laboratory studies almost always focus on tissues extracted from animals or on levels of blood components, such as hormones. Their findings are extremely remote from human beings with or without cancer and are difficult to apply to human survival. Though more directly applicable, most of the widely cited studies of humans are too small in scope, too short in length, and insufficiently definite in their measurement of psychological factors to provide much truly valuable information on the relationship between emotional health and cancer survival.

Debunking the Myth:
New Research Findings

Despite the weakness of pertinent research, many people still believe that patients who are emotionally distressed are more likely to die from cancer than those who are emotionally healthy. Patients, health professionals, and managers of health care delivery clearly require more definitive studies than most of those reported so far. Only improved studies can give patients accurate expectations, provide health professionals with good indications of the effectiveness of newly proposed treatments, and guide managers of health plans and medical practices in their selection of appropriate benefits for the seriously ill.

The best study of emotional factors in cancer survival would take the form of a clinical trial, akin to experiments that are standard in traditional biomedical research. In such a study, patients would be randomly assigned to different treatments—some, perhaps, to the Simonton method; others, to a traditional mode of treatment or a placebo situation, i.e., one known to be therapeutically neutral. As late as 1990, no such studies had been done.

Because scientists are reluctant to place people in randomized studies of unconventional treatment methods, clinical trials of emotionally based interventions may never take place. But investigations approximating the rigor of a clinical trial may provide better information than those usually cited in support of the emotional theory of survival. Studies of this kind must include several definite methods and procedures absent in the work reported earlier in this chapter.

First, these studies would have to be prospective. In prospective studies, researchers observe in advance the factors they expect to influence recovery or survival time. Such studies contrast with retrospective investigations, in which researchers locate survivors and attempt to assess their emotional well-being, or merely ask the survivors to explain their good fortune. Prospective studies require investigators to follow large numbers of patients over time. Many can be expected to die during the study. Prospective studies, however, lend themselves best to systematic comparison of survivors and nonsurvivors.

Next, the survivors and nonsurvivors compared in these studies must be similar in all respects other than the factors on which the researcher desires to focus—in this case, psychological health. In the event that an apparent relationship is found between emotional health and survival, the researcher must be able to rule out the possibility that other factors actually explain the result. For example, an apparent relationship between depression and poor survival chances may be explained by the plausible argument that patients with more advanced disease tend to experience more depression.

Third, a rigorous piece of research must use standardized measures of psychological factors. These include the extensive observational or paper-and-pencil tests familiar to most psychologists, such as the MMPI or SCL-90-R. These standard indicators keep investigators from consciously or unconsciously attributing to individual patients characteristics consistent with the favored hypothesis.

Fourth, a study with the required rigor must observe a fairly large number of patients. Studies of fewer than several hundred patients may fail to detect important relationships. Even where a relationship *does* exist between a measure of psychological well-being and survival, for example, a smaller number of observations may not support statistical significance. It is important to remember that statistical significance means that an observed relationship is unlikely to have occurred by chance.

Finally, a rigorous study must include clear hypotheses that specify the expected relationship between variables of interest. In the present context, these variables would include psychological factors such as stress, depression, inability to express oneself, lack of social adjustment, and other difficulties. These factors would be used to predict an outcome such as recovery from disease or extended survival time. The classical scientific tradition holds that researchers must be able to test hypotheses by systematically observing facts.

A RIGOROUS INVESTIGATION
OF PSYCHOLOGY AND SURVIVAL

Rigorous studies of the relationship between psychological well-being and cancer survival are just beginning to appear in scientific journals. One such study, nearly unique in its inclusion of the required features, was published in the *New England Journal of Medicine* in 1985.[19] Many physicians and scientists consider this journal the world's leading publication in biomedical research and medicine. In this study, University of Pennsylvania professor Barrie R. Cassileth and several of her colleagues observed 204 patients with cancers that were too advanced or rapidly spreading to warrant an attempt at surgery. They tested a series of hypotheses linking psychosocial factors and longevity. These researchers used thirty-two questions to measure various dimensions of psychological well-being or disturbance, including strength of social ties and marital history, job satisfaction, use of psychotropic drugs, general satisfaction with life, subjective view of health, helplessness and lack of hope, and perceived difficulty in adjusting to a diagnosis of life-threatening disease. All questions used were drawn from earlier studies by established researchers, and thus represented standard means of measuring psychological distress.

The Cassileth study was prospective. Patients were recruited for study during stays at the University of Pennsylvania hospital and were interviewed shortly after diagnosis of cancer. In many important respects, the patients were quite similar. Eligibility for the study included a strict and narrow set of disease characteristics, precluding the mixture of likely survivors and persons facing near-term mortality. Clinical factors such as site of the cancer, extent of the disease, and treatment received, moreover, were not statistically related to the psychological variables. The absence of such a relationship strongly suggests that patients with "good" versus "bad" psychological test outcomes differed *only* on the psychological variables themselves. Patients were followed until they died or for up to five years after their diagnoses.

This landmark study found no relationship between emotional well-being and survival. None of the relationships between the psychological variables tested and survival was statistically significant. Only familiar biological variables, such as extent of disease and limitations on physical functioning (probably related to the organic disease process), predicted early death.

Individual studies are never definitive. Cassileth herself recognizes that psychological factors may play a more important role in the survival of persons with more favorable prognoses. Most of the patients in her study were essentially incurable. Critics carped at the measures used by Cassileth, arguing that larger numbers of questions must be used to assess each individual psychological dimension. Noting the limitations of the measures used in the Cassileth study, one group of critics comments: "In their belief that psychosocial factors can be adequately represented by seven poor measures, the authors ignore the dynamic richness and variety of human experience."[20]

The conviction that psychological well-being improves survival chances is difficult to shake. Believers in the theory of course question the Cassileth findings. The research issues are indeed complex and require additional, confirmatory studies with the same rigor as Cassileth's study, using alternative means of psychological measurement. The SLACS provided an opportunity for such an investigation.

EMOTIONS AND CANCER SURVIVAL: THE SLACS FINDINGS

The SLACS provides an unusually detailed look at cancer patients. Based on a survey of 536 individuals, it encompasses a larger number of cases than most psychosocial investigations. Through extensive face-to-face interviews, the researchers were able to obtain vast amounts of reliable data on the lives, problems, and psychosocial well-being or distress of these patients. The resulting accumulation of data enabled the investigators to perform a study of psychological factors in survival that was more rigorous than perhaps any conducted in the past. Moreover, they were able to follow individual patients for up to eighty months, reinterviewing many on several occasions to monitor important changes in life conditions and outlook. All patients were followed for at least five years.

The SLACS included a long series of questions designed to measure psychological well-being. One particularly useful set of measures was the Profile of Mood States, or POMS. The POMS uses sixty-five individual questions to measure a series of variables similar to those examined by Cassileth: tension, depression, anger, confusion, fatigue, and vigor. Groups of individual questions are combined to generate indices of these variables, a process substantially reducing measurement error. Specialists in measurement of psychological variables have repeatedly examined the POMS for reliability and validity, confirming that persons taking the POMS respond the same way in repeated administrations and that the individual indices—tension, depression, etc.—measure the characteristics their names suggest. The POMS is particularly useful since it has been employed in several studies of cancer patients.

To assess the impacts of psychological well-being versus distress on survival, the SLACS investigators used each of the POMS scales as independent variables. They focused on two dependent variables reflecting mortality risk. First, they examined five-year survival. For statistical comparison, researchers often consider cancer patients who survive five years after diagnosis to be "cured." Second, they assessed the relative mortality risk of people with differing scores on each of the POMS measures—that is, the ratio of mortality risk (over the entire course of the study) among patients with higher-level POMS scores versus mortality risk among patients with lower-level POMS scores. While less familiar than five-year survival, relative risk is sometimes more important. This variable is more closely related to the length of time patients may be expected to live after diagnosis. Among persons with aggressive forms of cancer, methods of extending life for limited periods of time may be more important than attempts at cure as traditionally defined.

The researchers used statistical procedures that took account of important characteristics, other than emotional states, that may also have affected an individual patient's survival chances. These variables included age, sex, and the key disease features, cancer site and stage. Details of this analysis appear in Appendix B.

Figure 5 summarizes the results of this analysis, comparing five-year survival among individuals with differing score ranges on individual dimensions of the POMS. Persons with low numerical scores on an individual POMS dimension (e.g., "Tension") are considered free of noticeable symptoms or pathology on that dimension; in Figure 5, their symptom level is designated as "none." The symptoms of persons with middle-range scores are characterized as "slight"; those of persons with high scores are characterized as "extreme." To evaluate the possibility that differences presented in Figure 5 were observed by mere chance, levels of statistical significance were computed. In computing statistical significance, the researchers compared percentages of five-year survivors in the "none" category with percentages of five-year survivors in the "slight" and "extreme" categories.

The percentages appearing in Figure 5 are not direct observations. They are adjusted for differences in survival that may be traced to factors other than scores on the POMS—factors such as the patient's sex, age, and cancer site or stage. Computations for this chapter combine cancers of the lung, pancreas, prostate, and cervix.

Figure 5 presents no evidence that an individual's level of tension, depression, or anger makes a life-or-death difference. None of the relationships of anger, tension, or depression to five-year survival is large

Emotional distress does not predict survival.

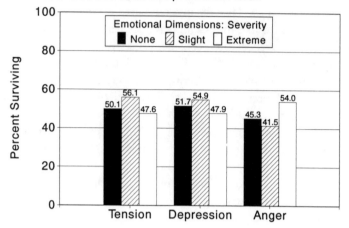

But physical symptoms do predict survival.

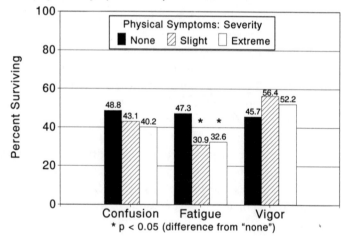

* p < 0.05 (difference from "none")

Fig. 5. *Emotional distress, physical symptoms, and five-year survival rates.*

enough to rule out the likelihood that it was observed by chance. Percentages of five-year survivors in the categories designating "slight" and "extreme" symptoms, moreover, are sometimes higher than in the category labeled "none." The pattern—or, rather, the absence of a pattern—linking these POMS dimensions with relative mortality risk is highly similar.

Figure 5 presents a more consistent set of findings based on the POMS dimensions of confusion, fatigue, and vigor. In comparison with individuals who show no discernible levels of confusion or fatigue, those with slight or extreme levels have poorer chances of five-year survival. Less vigorous people have lower chances of five-year survival. The figures include statistically significant differences on the dimension of fatigue. Statistics computed for relative mortality risk follow a highly similar pattern.

Some may view these findings as support for the position that psychological well-being indeed promotes cancer survival. But a closer look at the measures casts doubt on such a conclusion. Although the six dimensions measured by the POMS are *intended* to reflect "mood states," only half of them really indicate emotional phenomena. Tension, depression, and anger are clearly emotional dimensions. Strong arguments can be made, however, that confusion, fatigue, and vigor actually reflect *physical phenomena.* These three terms do not sound truly psychological. Research has demonstrated, moreover, that indices with the latter three titles in the POMS correlate strongly with other disease symptoms and physical dysfunction among the seriously ill.[21] It appears essential to view the POMS Tension, Depression, and Anger indices as measuring perhaps related but different phenomena from the Confusion, Fatigue, and Vigor indicators.

When viewed with this distinction in mind, Figure 5 provides no indication that emotional distress affects cancer survival. The relationships that do appear in Figure 5 are easily explained as the consequence of physical disease. Cancer patients who report that they are extraordinarily tired (indicated by "fatigue" and "vigor") are likely to be sicker, and hence more likely to die in the near term, than those who are physically less ill. The confused patient could well be taking pain-killing or mood-altering drugs.

Other measures in the SLACS also cast doubt on the psychological theory. Two indices from the widely used Sickness Impact Profile (SIP)[22] showed no relationship with either five-year survival or relative mortality risk. One index, built from nine separate questions, measured "emotional behavior," a composite of such adverse feelings as self-blame and hopelessness. The other index, comprising twenty separate questions, measured impaired social interaction resulting from illness; individual questions touched on loss of humor, withdrawal of affection, self-isolation, and the like. Many health researchers consider marriage a reflection of emotional stability and a cause of positive adjustment and feelings. Married people observed in this study, however, had no survival advantage, beyond what might have been observed by chance, over those who were not married.

Finally, the SLACS detected no evidence that the patient's mood state deteriorates with the approach of death. Patients with the most aggressive forms of cancer (lung and pancreatic) were interviewed every two to three months, and this process was repeated as many times as possible before the patients became too ill or died. Among these patients, average levels of tension, depression, and anger tended to remain constant over the successive interviews. The consistency of these observations has two implications. First, it suggests that a single measure of mood state soon after diagnosis is a good reflection of the patient's general feelings over time. A specialist in measurement might conclude that the POMS reflects not just emotional "state" but long-term "trait." Second, the view over time confirms the impression from Figure 5 that psychological distress does not, in general, foreshadow death.

IMPLICATIONS OF SLACS FINDINGS

For professionals and patients concerned with obtaining an accurate, objective assessment of the relationship between emotions and cancer survival, the Cassileth study and the SLACS represent crucial sources of information. Because these studies observe large numbers of patients and follow each individual prospectively to monitor his or her survival, they differ markedly from the investigations usually cited by supporters of the emotional theory of survival. Perhaps alone among studies of emotional factors and cancer survival, these two investigations used objective, quantitative measures of psychological variables. Both studies share the important feature of separating possible effects of disease and personal-background factors from the effects of psychological state. Clearly, the Cassileth study and the SLACS come closer to the rigors of traditional science than most other investigations of the psychosocial aspects of cancer. Neither of these two powerful studies provides evidence that the patient's emotional state affects his or her chances for survival in any way.

Devotees of the emotional theory of cancer survival often cite Hans Selye as the founder of their approach. He was one of the most important of the modern physicians who have studied the relationship between stress and illness, publishing studies in this area as far back as 1936. Authors of influential books on the relation of emotions and behavior to heart disease draw upon Selye's contributions; writers on Type A and Type B behavior, for instance, usually refer to Selye's pioneering work. Simonton, Cousins, and other popular authors look to Selye for evidence on the relation between emotional well-being and cancer survival.

Selye, however, was extremely cautious about explaining cancer on the basis of emotions and behavior. Reviewing a vast quantity of research findings shortly before his own death, Selye pointed out that, while stress produced some hormonal responses that might produce cancer growth, stress could produce responses that *inhibited* such growth as well. Summarizing the research, he concluded that "a certain predisposition is necessary in all . . . maladies, and the same is true of cancer, in which the role of stress has been extensively studied, but is still far from clear."[23]

Selye was even more cautious about the benefits of psychiatric and behavioral interventions intended to prolong the lives of cancer patients. He wrote:

Considerable literature has accumulated concerning the relationship between cancer and the mind. The interpretation of most of the reports is extremely difficult and subject to doubt. It has even been claimed that, under certain conditions, neoplasms can result from psychosomatic reactions in that certain predisposing personality characteristics and emotional states may play a significant role in the development, site, and course of cancer. On the other hand, regression of malignancies as a consequence of the patient's strong will to survive has also been postulated, but there is little tangible evidence to support such a view. Perhaps the most pressing task in this connection is to develop a code of behavior among patients with incurable malignancies and to train medical personnel in the techniques of making these trying times as tolerable as possible to the patients and to their relatives.[24]

Anecdotes cited as evidence for a connection between emotions and cancer survival, moreover, might be very different if the lives of their subjects were followed for any length of time. It would be useful to monitor the lives of patients of Simonton and others in the therapeutic movement he represents. How long do the enthusiastic, positive-sounding patients receiving this form of care actually survive? How typical is the fate of a SLACS patient who died soon after giving this enthusiastic testimony: "I went to the doctor to ask about pain under my ribs. I was given X rays, waited two days for the results, and then was rushed to emergency surgery. I couldn't breathe. The doctor said it was a malignant tumor. Everyone prayed—and at the surgery, they never found it. The Lord had removed the tumor—there was no trace."

◆   ◆   ◆   ◆   ◆

In the late twentieth century, two approaches to the cancer problem outside the realm of orthodox medicine became quite popular. The first asserted that preventive measures could solve most of the cancer problem. The second alleged that favorable emotions and attitudes could reduce cancer mortality. Both approaches appealed to the basic American value that people can attain the most difficult goals by adopting the proper attitudes and taking action on their own behalf. Both could well have reflected frustration with the slow rate of progress medicine seemed to be making in pursuit of a cure for cancer. Both appear to stem from cultural support for individual initiative, exaggeration of fundamentally sound theory and facts, and perhaps wishful thinking.

As late as the 1990s, the few rigorous investigations of the relation between psychological factors and cancer survival indicated no potential benefit from interventions addressing the patient's emotional state. Researchers, practitioners, and policymakers should continue to seek ways outside the strictly technical offerings of medicine to increase cancer survival. A better understanding of the part played by human thinking, behavior, and conditions of life may indeed suggest important new steps to be taken. But the most promising approaches to reducing cancer mortality outside the traditional thinking of biology and medicine appear likely to involve areas other than the individual patient's attitude, personality, or mood.

CHAPTER SIX

Early Detection:
The Key to Cancer Survival?

Of all defenses against cancer, early detection is by far the most familiar. Early cancer detection requires both effective medical technology and appropriate human behavior. To detect cancer while it is still localized and presumably easiest to treat, physicians must possess appropriate skills and equipment. But early detection also appears to represent a nonbiomedical factor in cancer survival. The process depends on appropriate patient behavior: individuals initiating contact with the health care system in the absence of gross or long-standing symptoms. For a physician or clinic, successful early detection serves as an indication of high-quality care, combining medical technology with effective patient motivation and access to services.

This chapter examines the role that early detection may play in improving a patient's prospects for surviving cancer. The familiarity of early detection as a method of improving cancer survival does not mean that it actually works as many believe. As the preceding chapter has shown, popular beliefs about health and illness are often inaccurate. Emphasis on early detection to promote cancer survival has, in fact, much in common with the beliefs that most cancers can be prevented and that psychological health may lead to a cancer cure. Almost every American has heard and supports the assertion that cancer can be cured if it is caught early. Under careful examination, will this belief, too, prove a myth?

Taking effective steps to improve cancer survival requires a critical examination of early detection. A strong case can be made for early detection on the basis of the most elementary facts about cancer. A cancer detected early in its natural history, it would appear, should remain confined to a limited area, accessible to the surgeon's knife. Yet some scientists, armed with detailed knowledge of cancer and its development, contend that early detection has received more attention than it deserves. Important research findings, in fact, provide a basis for the conclusion that early detection is often useless in curing cancer, and perhaps even harmful to some cancer patients.

This chapter attempts to provide a balanced view of early detection. It reviews claims, familiar at least in concept to most, that have been made for the importance of early detection. It summarizes some of the key studies and arguments—likely new knowledge to most nonspecialists—that question the value of early detection. As in the evaluation of emotional factors in cancer survival, the SLACS adds new information useful in assessing the value of early detection.

The Case for Early Detection

The basic argument for early detection rests on the principle that cancer cells tend to multiply rapidly and give rise to tumors in places beyond their points of origin. The common feature of all cancer cells may be that, despite this tendency toward proliferation, they cannot perform the vital functions of normal cells. Some cancers may remain locally invasive, forming masses only in the tissues where they originate. Others spread beyond the area of origin through the blood or lymph systems. More extensive growth corresponds to more serious disease. Even if tumors remain at their sites of origin, they may interfere with vital body functions as they become larger. The seeding of tumor cells in distant organs creates potential for similar problems in many locations, making surgery and radiation less definitive forms of therapy.

Early detection, it is presumed, benefits the patient by allowing treatment to begin early in the disease process, before dissemination of malignant cells becomes extensive. Localized disease, it would appear, is more easily cured. Thus, minimizing the time between the appearance of the first abnormal cell and initiation of treatment should give the patient a better chance to survive.

The American Cancer Society has been perhaps the strongest advocate for early detection. As early as 1913, leaders of the American Society for the Control of Cancer, the precursor of the American Cancer Society, had begun publishing pamphlets and magazine articles urging people to see their doctors at the slightest hint of trouble. Armed with new leadership and vastly increased financial resources, the American Cancer Society intensified its efforts to promote early detection in the 1940s and 1950s. Nearly every American who could read became acquainted with cancer's "seven danger signals": any sore that does not heal; a lump or thickening in the breast or elsewhere; unusual bleeding or discharge; any change in a wart or mole; persistent indigestion or difficulty in swallowing; persistent hoarseness or cough; any change in normal bowel habits. Along with advocacy for increased cancer research, messages stressing the urgency of early detection have constituted the most consistent themes of the American Cancer Society throughout its history. The society's messages became so powerful that even some who agreed with them in substance began to caution that the fear they engendered might cause people to deny symptoms and actually avoid early detection.[1]

Publicity to encourage early detection remained a major American Cancer Society program into the late 1980s. In 1987, an American Cancer Society publication projected that 483,000 Americans would die of cancer in that year and suggested that 35 percent of the expected mortality (or about 170,000 people) could be prevented through early detection.[2]

In the mid-twentieth century, new tools for early detection encouraged advocates of this approach to cancer survival. Procedures capable of detecting early-stage cancers of the uterine cervix, breast, and colon came into widespread use in this period. In 1987, cancers of the colon and rectum accounted for about 11 percent of cancer deaths among American men. Cervical, breast, and colon cancers were responsible for about one-third of the cancer deaths among American women in that year.

The Pap test is the best example of a method of early cancer detection in use today. The test is named after Dr. George Papanicolaou, who spearheaded its development in the 1930s and 1940s. It is a simple and inexpensive procedure for early detection of cervical cancer. To perform the Pap test, a health practitioner collects cells from the patient's cervix by scraping with a swab. This procedure may take place in a variety of settings, including doctors' offices, hospitals, and clinics. Later, a technician examines the cells under a microscope to detect evidence of disease. Although the procedure may cause some discomfort, it is quick and safe.

The Pap test is most useful in detecting changes in cervical tissue that may foreshadow the development of cancer. In cancer of the cervix, as in several other malignancies, normal tissues develop distinguishing characteristics which indicate that the tissues may later become malignant. Patients with these findings must undergo biopsies to determine the exact nature of their condition. Many physicians now use a magnifying device called a colposcope to locate actual areas of abnormality and thus minimize the amount of tissue removed in biopsy or treatment.[3] This device is particularly helpful in safeguarding fertility in women of child-bearing age.

Early detection of cervical cancer through the Pap test is apparently valuable in improving chances for survival. In the years following introduction of the Pap test, mortality from cervical cancer declined steadily—especially in countries that have aggressively used the Pap test as a public health measure. The Scandinavian countries provide a useful comparison. Because these countries are strong welfare states, their populations encounter few if any economic barriers to medical care. In Sweden, where a cervical cancer screening program has been in operation, advanced-stage cervical cancer has declined markedly.[4] In Norway, however, which has lacked a vigorous cervical cancer screening program, rates of advanced cervical cancer have declined more slowly.[5]

Breast cancer, in the opinion of many experts, is also amenable to early detection. Mammography, perhaps the best-known technique for early detection, is a low-dose X ray capable of detecting nonpalpable tumors, those too small to be found in a physical examination. Thermography, a related technique, distinguishes subtle variations in heat radiated from the breast, facilitating detection of tumors without using potentially hazardous X rays.

Proponents of early detection often cite a study of mammography in the 1960s and 1970s as a major milestone. The study took place at the Health Insurance Plan (HIP) of Greater New York, a pioneering health maintenance organization (HMO) with over 500,000 members. In the HIP study, 31,000 randomly selected women were offered mammographic examinations at their medical group centers, and were asked to return for three annual follow-up examinations. A control group of 31,000 women was identified, but these women were allowed to follow normal patterns of medical care. The researchers followed both groups for nine years in order to compare death rates. Women in the mammography group experienced a one-third reduction in mortality from breast cancer compared with the controls.[6]

Breast self-examination is another widely noted technique for early detection of breast cancer. In addition to regular mammograms, the American Cancer Society and other authorities recommend that women periodically examine their own breasts for lumps or other suspicious signs. Most breast cancer patients detect their own tumors. Educational literature is available to instruct women in the most effective techniques of breast self-examination and encourage them to perform the procedure regularly.

Finally, early detection of colon and rectal cancer has received much attention. Because these malignancies tend to develop slowly and have definite precursor conditions (growths called polyps in the colon or rectum), early detection appears likely to allow treatment not only at an early stage but even before the cancer develops. Patients with early colon and rectal cancers have much better survival chances than those with later-stage disease. Testing for blood in the stool has shown great promise for aiding early detection. The 1980s saw commercial availability of simple devices for detecting blood in the stool invisible to the naked eye. Such tests for occult blood take the form of slides impregnated with chemicals that react to traces of blood in characteristic ways. Many of these tests can be self-administered, then sent back to physicians' offices or read by the patient.

Other methods widely used to detect colorectal cancer at an early stage include the digital rectal examination and sigmoidoscopy. The digital rectal exam is an old, straightforward procedure but is capable of detecting lesions only as far into the large bowel as the physician's finger can reach. With the aid of a sigmoidoscope, a fiber-optic device for scanning the lower portion of the colon, the physician can detect 40 to 50 percent of all colorectal cancers. In one study carried out in Minnesota between 1946 and 1979, 18,000 patients were screened with sigmoidoscopy and thirteen cancers were detected, all localized. None of those found to have cancer had died by 1979. The number of cancers detected was far below those expected to occur, perhaps because polyps detected in the sigmoidoscopy were removed.[7] A New York study carried out over fifteen years, involving 26,000 subjects, detected fifty malignancies; 90 percent of those with cancer survived until the conclusion of the study.[8]

At this point, it is important to distinguish the process of *screening* from that of *early detection*. Screening is a preliminary step in the early-detection process. Screening does not result in diagnosis of cancer, but identifies signs possibly indicating cancer among individuals in an apparently well population. When appropriately used, positive findings in a screening procedure lead to further investigation by health professionals, typically involving more intensive examination—for example, colonoscopy following a positive occult fecal blood test, or biopsy for nearly all conditions. No true early detection, however, can take place solely on the basis of screening. There is no true early detection without definitive diagnosis.

Most of the early-detection methods discussed here are, in fact, screening procedures. As such, they could fit into either public health screening programs or routine examinations given by physicians to their regular patients. The Pap test and occult fecal blood detection share characteristics identified by specialists as most desirable for screening procedures.[9] They address diseases that occur frequently in the community. They are simple, accurate, reliable, and acceptable to large numbers of patients. They are inexpensive. They are capable of helping detect diseases for which treatment exists. Perhaps most important, they involve diseases that have a distinct detectable preclinical phase, during which physicians can effectively intervene but in which minimum disease dissemination or loss of function takes place.

While logically interconnected, screening and diagnosis frequently are separate activities, taking place in different locations and carried out by different personnel. Advocates of early detection have taken vastly differing approaches to the linkage between these two components. In its post–World War II literature, the American Cancer Society seemed to consider the physician's office an appropriate site for both screening and diagnosis; its literature consistently emphasized the slogan "Every Doctor's Office a Cancer Detection Center."[10] At mid-century, advocates of early detection established free-standing, multiphasic screening centers in several major cities. Centers such as the Strang Clinic in New York, the Fox-Chase Clinic in Philadelphia, and the Portes Center in Chicago specialized in cancer screening only, separate from diagnosis and treatment. At these centers, patients—or "screenees," as they were more accurately called—were run through sequences of screening procedures for the most common cancers. In another break with traditional health care, procedures could be entirely automated, as was a computerized health history station at the Portes Center. In the event of positive findings, "screenees" were advised to consult their physicians for further evaluation and care.

If the word *cancer* engenders fear, the term *early detection* suggests hope. In the popular mind as well in the thinking of many professionals, early detection helps transform cancer from a sure killer to a manageable risk, controllable through scientific means. Solid factual evidence and advances in clinical medicine seem to support this thinking. Cancer in perhaps all its forms appears less lethal if diagnosed in an early stage. Technologies such as the Pap test and mammography—whose application may take place outside traditional medical practice—seem to represent meaningful progress in achieving early detection for larger and larger numbers of people.

The Limits of Early Detection

Enthusiastic as most are about early detection, it is surprising to learn that some scientists and health professionals voice serious reservations about its benefits. Early detection, some caution, often has no real power to extend the lives of those who contract cancer. In an age when health care costs receive so much attention, some critics suggest that resources now used to detect cancer early might be better employed elsewhere. Others warn that the process of early detection and treatment, cost notwithstanding, can cause the patient significant harm. Moreover, problems in real-life application may limit the benefits of early detection, despite the concept's appeal.

CLINICAL CONCERNS

The fact that cancer comprises a large number of diseases with vastly different characteristics limits the effectiveness of early detection in promoting survival. All cancers may involve the development of cell masses that cannot perform normal biological functions and spread beyond their points of origin. But apart from this common denominator, malignancies differ markedly in detectability and aggressiveness—the speed with which they grow and their range of dissemination throughout the body. Furthermore, physicians do not have equal success in arresting the growth of all types of cancer cells. The slogan "Cancer can be cured if it is caught early" is much more true for some forms of the disease than for others.

Pancreatic cancer represents a stark contrast to, say, cancer of the uterine cervix. As of the mid-1980s, no screening procedures were available for pancreatic cancer among individuals without symptoms. Certain signs may lead a physician to suspect pancreatic cancer: weight loss, pain, jaundice, a family history. But diagnosis and evaluation for eventual treatment require at the very least a sampling of bile or pancreatic juices. Because procedures for obtaining such specimens require passing instruments deep inside the body, they are not used on patients who are apparently well. When pancreatic cancer is suspected, the patient may have to undergo surgery, so that the type and extent of disease can be evaluated before definitive treatment is attempted. Even then, the physician may not know what the patient really has. As one authority commented recently on the difficulties surrounding knowledge about pancreatic cancer, "Half the diagnoses may be wrong, and at autopsy examination, half the cases of pancreatic cancer are unexpected."[11] While cancers occurring in some parts of the pancreas readily cause pain and may thus encourage physicians to use these diagnostic procedures, those occurring in other parts of the organ often remain "silent" until they have undergone significant growth.

With respect to benefits obtainable through early detection, lung cancer seems to fall between cancers of the cervix and pancreas. Current screening tests and diagnostic procedures for lung cancer have the characteristics necessary to encourage their use on patients without symptoms: low cost, little inconvenience, and minor risk. X rays, for instance, can detect irregularities that may prove to be malignant lesions. Another procedure, sputum cytology, enables technicians and pathologists to examine a patient's sputum for the presence of cancer cells. The sputum cytology procedure can sometimes detect cancers that are not flagged by X rays.

In lung cancer, the impact of early detection on survival is uncertain. Researchers have conducted several extensive studies of the effectiveness of lung cancer screening. A study begun in 1971 at the Mayo Clinic compared 4,500 men in a special screening program with 4,500 others not in the program. All participants in the study were at high risk for lung cancer: over forty-five years of age and long-term tobacco smokers. Men in the screening program were encouraged to (1) have a chest X ray, (2) submit samples for sputum cytology, and (3) complete a health questionnaire every four months. The other men received only the Mayo Clinic's standard advice, to stop smoking and have a yearly health checkup with X ray and sputum cytology.[12]

Initial results proved hopeful. By the end of 1979, the researchers had detected more early-stage cases of lung cancer among men in the screening program than in the comparison group. But longer-term studies did not bear out the initial optimism. Neither the Mayo Clinic study nor similar investigations at Memorial Sloan-Kettering in New York and Johns Hopkins in Baltimore demonstrated that screening reduced mortality from lung cancer.[13] Reversing a position it had held earlier, the American Cancer Society in the early 1980s withdrew its recommendation of X-ray screening for persons at high risk for lung cancer.

Some evidence suggests that early detection of lung cancer may be beneficial, particularly if surer detection methods are developed. Authorities consider the prospects for survival of patients with some early-stage lung cancers to be excellent.[14] Today the vast majority of lung cancer patients obtain diagnoses with symptoms present, when significant spread is already likely to have occurred. But the nature of the disease itself may limit the potential benefits of any method of early detection. Observers have found that even lung cancer patients with early-stage disease, detected through aggressive screening, may have small, undetected tumors at the time of their surgery in addition to the growths actually removed. Malignant cells may begin to spread before the development of a visible initial tumor. Lung cancer may occur, moreover, in several different forms, some highly resistant to treatment even if caught early.

The benefits of early detection in prostate cancer are likewise uncertain. Most physicians include a digital rectal examination as part of the routine physical for older male patients, through which they readily detect enlargement of the prostate gland, which may signal cancer. The benign versus malignant status of such tumors may be established through a needle biopsy, which can be performed in the physician's office, or by examining tissue removed in a transurethral resection of the prostate (TURP), an operation that removes part of the enlarged gland to relieve urinary retention. Urologists often perform TURPs as therapy for enlarged prostates even when there is no suspicion of malignancy.

Physicians have not reached agreement on appropriate treatment for prostate cancer.[15] Uncertainty arises in part from the highly variable nature of the disease. Even in early-stage disease, some prostate cancers spread rapidly to surrounding tissues and bones, while others remain indolent for years. Physicians cannot always ascertain the "malignant potential" of localized prostate cancer through microscopic examination of the cells. Some physicians advocate extensive surgery, often alongside radiation therapy or use of hormones, to combat an early-stage cancer. Others treat conservatively or not at all, pointing out that many people who receive no treatment for this disease live on for years, while treatment exposes patients to dangerous side effects.

Even in diseases where most practitioners consider early detection beneficial, however, some analysts raise serious concerns. In one comprehensive study, a policy specialist and an epidemiologist question the usefulness and ultimate safety of the Pap test for individual women.[16] They note that several features of the test may lead to erroneous assessments of the danger of malignancy. Technicians inspecting a Papanicolaou-stained slide may fail to see evidence of abnormal tissue when it is in fact present in the woman from whom the sample was obtained—an error whose rate has been estimated as high as 20 percent. In other instances, suspicious findings on the Pap test may lead women to undergo surgical procedures such as hysterectomies unnecessarily. Science has not determined whether all tissues classified as "premalignant" become true cancers, with the capacity to invade other organs. Thus, many women may unnecessarily undergo the discomfort, cost, and side effects of surgery, including loss of fertility. Overall, cervical cancer may have declined not because of Pap testing but because of declines in social practices, such as prostitution, associated with the disease.

It is well demonstrated that screening does not improve chances of survival in all cancers. In some instances, technical capabilities for early detection do not exist. Detection of premalignant conditions may not foreshadow cancer but may cause some patients to undergo unnecessary treatments with attendant risks and side effects. Problems other than those associated with clinical-testing capabilities are visible as well.

PROBLEMS IN ORGANIZATION AND DELIVERY OF CARE

Good techniques for detecting cancer may fail because they are applied in a faulty manner. Some medical procedures in use today are clearly effective in detecting cancer at an early stage. But an individual walking into a doctor's office or screening center will not necessarily obtain the full benefits of such procedures—even if the patient has enough money or insurance to pay for early-detection services, the doctor's office or screening center has the right equipment, and all personnel are competent and well trained. Serious difficulties arise from the organization of services and the behavior of individual human beings.

The Risk of Technical Error. Technical errors that render potentially effective procedures useless may take place "behind the scenes." Sensitive cancer tests may be developed by brilliant scientists, but they must be carried out by ordinary mortals. Under the pressures and distractions of daily life, errors abound. Honest mistakes and deliberate corner-cutting occur everywhere, from the citizen filling out an income tax return to the assembly line worker welding an automobile part. Why not the laboratory technician scanning slides to distinguish normal cells from malignant ones?

Alarming reports of faulty management in cancer-detection laboratories have surfaced recently. Pap smear laboratory work constitutes an industry in itself, with workers handling specimens taken from millions of women every year. Focusing on the Pap smear, reporters from the *Wall Street Journal* visited laboratories, inspected records, and interviewed doctors, laboratory workers, and government officials. Highly disturbing conclusions in the newspaper's report (published on November 2, 1987) included the following: "What emerges is a picture of a Pap-screening industry kept afloat by over-worked, undersupervised, poorly paid technicians. It is an industry that often ignores what few laws protect women from slipshod testing."[17]

Across the nation, high-volume, cut-rate laboratories, sometimes called Pap factories or Pap mills, allow technicians to analyze up to four times as many specimens per year as medical experts recommend for accuracy. Many of them pay screeners on a piecework basis, which encourages the screeners to rush the analysis. The *Wall Street Journal*'s investigation uncovered the cases of several women whose Pap tests were misread, so that the women were given false assurance that they were cancer-free. Two of these women, aged thirty-four and thirty-six, died of invasive cervical cancer. A third, aged twenty-five, survived but became sterile as a result of the extensive treatment necessitated by late diagnosis.

According to this report, the need to process huge numbers of tests at low cost contributes significantly to the error rate. The processing of Pap tests requires skilled, conscientious human labor. Technicians must examine stained slides under a microscope, scanning thousands of cells taken from each individual woman to detect the few that may indicate cancer or conditions that may lead to cancer at a later time. In today's health care industry, which stresses cost restraint, many doctors and health plans send specimens to the laboratories that offer the lowest rates, but do not always offer adequate assurance of quality.

While qualified technicians must have college degrees plus additional training, they may earn as little as forty-five cents per Pap test slide. This infinitesimal remuneration encourages them to scan slides rapidly if they are paid on a piecework basis or, if they are paid on salary, to hurry through quotas at one laboratory in order to take second and third jobs at other facilities. In 1987, only one state (California) had laws limiting the number of slides a technician could read in a single day—and the law was often violated. It is a common practice for technicians to take slides home and examine them there, without direct supervision, and often in the presence of family distractions.

Regulation of individual proficiency also appears weak. Federal laws apply to Pap testing only if it is performed under Medicare or if the laboratory is in interstate commerce. States license laboratories and have powers of inspection. In 1987, however, only New York State required technicians to pass proficiency tests in screening Pap smear slides. Voluntary professional organizations, such as the College of American Pathologists and the American Society of Cytology, offer certification to laboratories that can meet their criteria, and doctors concerned with quality often look to such certification. But, according to the *Wall Street Journal*, many of the largest labs have never sought accreditation.

Physicians themselves must share some of the responsibility for the Pap test's failure to yield its maximum benefits for cancer survival. According to comments from several leading cancer specialists, half the incorrect results of Pap testing arise from the physician's collecting inadequate cell samples. Efforts to educate physicians to take better specimens have often been unsuccessful. According to a past president of the American Cancer Society, moreover, "even good labs" are reluctant to reject inadequate slides sent to them (which might encourage physicians to improve) for fear of losing business.

It would be a serious error to assume that these problems occur with every cancer test, in every laboratory, and in every medical practice. However, the Pap test is one of the few cancer-screening procedures almost universally acknowledged as beneficial. Even in a well-established technical procedure, improper application can weaken benefits for the population and cause tragedy in individual lives. Other problems in the application of proven cancer-detection technology may be equally serious.

The Lessons of Automated Screening. Early detection may promote cancer survival only insofar as related health services are effectively organized. To recapitulate, the organization of care encompasses the complex sets of human relations involved in the provision of services: relationships among different health care professionals; between groups of health professionals; between those providing health care and insurance companies or the government; between the providers and consumers of services. Even if all medical procedures for early detection were carried out flawlessly, survival would not be increased to its full potential if organization were faulty.

Automated screening, a concept that gained favor in the 1950s and persisted through the rest of the twentieth century, illustrates some of the problems with early detection that may reduce the benefits obtainable through proven technical means. This procedure makes use of a package of the low-cost, high-volume cancer-screening tests that have been individually hailed as valuable public health measures. "Automation" in this connection reflects a highly standardized cancer-detection procedure, involving relatively little human intervention or decision-making during the screening process itself. This automated procedure illustrates the possibility that too great a separation of screening from actual diagnosis and treatment may make early detection less effective.

A study in the 1970s of a specialized cancer-screening facility in the Midwest provides an example.[18] The "Metropolitan Screening Center" (a fictitious name) offered an extensive battery of tests, including most standardized cancer-detection procedures, such as X rays, proctoscopy, and mammography. Screening began with a health history, the patient reading questions on a computer screen and responding on the keyboard. The patient then moved from station to station in a preprogrammed sequence of tests, concluding with an examination by a physician and a counseling session. The entire process took about three hours and cost $80 in 1977.

The screening center enjoyed a favorable reputation in the locality and retained a loyal group of patients, who returned for screening every year. But the study revealed that another group of patients clearly did not receive the maximum benefits the screening procedures offered, because they failed to take follow-up actions. The center provided neither definitive diagnosis nor treatment. Instead, patients were told by the center's physicians, both in face-to-face counseling sessions and by letter, that they should immediately consult their own physicians about any suspicious indications found in the screening. But nearly 25 percent of patients who were so informed did not act on the center's advice for four months or longer. About 16 percent of those in whom a possible indication of cancer was detected never took *any* action. For these individuals, advantages gained from early detection at the center were reduced if not entirely lost because of delay or inaction.

Factors related both to the characteristics of the patients and to the center's style of operation contributed to this inaction. In interviews, many of those who failed to act explained that they had been afraid to find out whether they actually had cancer. But fear is probably not the whole explanation. Fear is a very reasonable and widespread response to the possibility of cancer. Doubtless, many of those who took prompt action did so despite their fear.

Differing experiences with the broader health care system seemed to distinguish those who took prompt action from those who delayed. Patients who had strong preexisting ties to providers outside the Metropolitan Screening Center were the quickest to take action when informed of suspicious findings. Typically, these people had named regular physicians on the center's intake forms, suggesting that they had established relations with professionals they could turn to when problems arose. Many, including some without regular doctors, seemed to share an attitude reflecting confidence in the broader health care system. These people indicated that they went to the screening center as part of a periodic routine to maintain good health. Those who hesitated to seek medical follow-up or took no action at all evidenced weaker relations to the broader system and less favorable attitudes toward it. Interviews with these people revealed that several had attempted to establish relations with "good family doctors" but had been unable to do so—either because they had only recently moved to the city, or because their family doctor had retired or died, or because they were unable to locate an acceptable neighborhood practice. Two inner-city dwellers, for example, characterized available medical services in their neighborhoods as "Medicaid mills." Among those who delayed obtaining follow-up or took no action, several seemed particularly alienated from physicians, blaming them for the deaths of relatives and characterizing them as "robber barons" and "rip-off artists."

In addition to the relationships of patients to the broader health care system, characteristics of the screening center itself seemed to affect follow-up action. The automated, sometimes cold-seeming nature of the Metropolitan Screening Center seemed to reinforce preexisting negative experiences with the health care system in several instances. Several of those who delayed said that they felt "like an object going down an assembly line" and "just like a slab of meat." Expecting an improvement over services they had received in the broader health care system, these patients were disappointed. In their overall experience, a vicious cycle of successively deeper alienation seems to have occurred, which greatly reduced their benefits from the center's technical capabilities.

These observations illustrate the limitations that behavioral and organizational factors may place on even technically proven methods for detecting cancer. In the Metropolitan Screening Center, a combination of "high tech" and "low touch" appears likely to have caused at least some patients to delay or never initiate follow-up of suspicious findings. But even in health care settings more traditional than the Metropolitan Screening Center, delay in diagnosis or treatment may have little to do with the qualities or actions of the patient.

System-Related Causes of Delay. Both health care professionals and the systems within which they work may contribute to delay in diagnosing and treating cancer. Several researchers have focused on physician behavior as a cause of delay. As long ago as the 1930s, a researcher reported that, about one-third of the time, physicians were partially or completely responsible for delay in cancer diagnosis. In these instances, delay resulted from the physician's failure to make a diagnosis or refer the patient elsewhere within one month of the first visit.[19] Focusing on practice settings, later researchers reported that factors such as method of payment, lack of convenient laboratory facilities, and referral to distantly located consultants contributed to delay in initiating definitive treatment.[20]

In any major medical center—with its technical sophistication, physical size, and organizational complexity—opportunities for malfunctions abound, even when the center is staffed by personnel of the highest competency and dedication. X rays and laboratory tests may be faultily performed. Reports from such procedures may get lost. Scheduling routines may override clinical urgency. Minor equipment malfunctions may delay important procedures. The degree to which these and similar factors delay or reduce the efficacy of early detection and contribute to preventable mortality is unknown.

Of equal concern is the possibility that today's health care providers may have deliberate policies that result in delaying cancer detection or treatment. Because physicians and hospitals alike face increasing pressure to control costs, physicians may make less aggressive use of screening tests. Health care facilities that receive advance payments for all patient services—an increasingly widespread payment mechanism—may reduce laboratory or surgery facilities and employ or contract with fewer of the specialists required to make definitive diagnoses or carry out treatment. In such instances, patients may have to wait longer for detection, treatment, or both. Anecdotes told about the British National

Health Service underscore these concerns. It is said that this system has mandated a year-long waiting period for coronary bypass surgery (readily available in the United States), on the assumption that some candidates will die during the interim, reducing demand for the operation and thus costs. Experts in health service delivery recognize that such waiting periods are a form of rationing. Many in the United States believe that such rationing is beginning to take place here with increasing frequency, although few advocate it openly as a means of cutting costs.

Early Detection and Survival in Three Cancers

While most health professionals and laypeople believe in early cancer detection, several major questions arise about this approach to cancer survival. Some of these questions concern the nature of cancer in general and the characteristics of individual malignancies. How many types of cancer may actually be detected early enough for available therapies to make a difference in survival? At the point where a person notices one of the danger signs of cancer, how often has the disease progressed too far for even immediate treatment to make survival more likely? Other questions address the actual process by which cancer is detected. How important are steps initiated by patients (e.g., response to a cancer warning sign) in comparison with steps taken by providers of health care (such as scheduling for treatment following a cancer diagnosis)?

The SLACS helps answer some of these questions as they apply to lung, prostate, and cervical cancer. Although the SLACS also included pancreatic cancer, this disease has been omitted from consideration in the present chapter and in Chapters 7 and 8. These chapters address behavioral and service delivery issues that did not apply well to pancreatic cancer, given the major technical limitations that prevailed in detection and treatment of this malignancy at the time the study was conducted.

To learn more about the early-detection process, the researchers asked patients how their malignancies had been detected and diagnosed. They examined information from medical records to delve further into this process. Most important, they followed the patients over the years to learn the connections between aspects of the detection process and the outcome of cancer treatment—namely, survival versus death.

Limitations in previous work by scientists concerned with early detection made this research necessary. Like the studies described above, most research has concentrated on the technical features of early detection. Studies of mammography for breast cancer, sigmoidoscopy for colon cancer, and sputum cytology for lung cancer have usually tested the effectiveness of the techniques themselves—the machines, the laboratory tests, the physical examination procedures. These studies, for example, compare patients undergoing newly developed screening tests with patients not undergoing such procedures. In making this comparison, researchers attempt to determine whether the randomly selected experimental subjects (those who are tested) are diagnosed earlier in the course of the disease and live longer. But in the real world, successful early detection requires more than proven medical techniques.

Even the most important early-detection studies shed little light on questions of human behavior and the organization of care. The landmark Health Insurance Plan (HIP) of Greater New York breast cancer–screening study provides an example.[21] The HIP is a large prepaid health plan. Conducting the study on its members, most of whom, in the mid-1960s, received coverage as a benefit from work, the researchers were unable to evaluate the importance of individual initiative. Working people who join an HMO may be especially likely to take personal responsibility for their well-being. The experimental setup itself generated repeated communication with the patients, to encourage regular examinations. The HMO, moreover, provided any needed care at no additional charge. The thinking, habits, and resources of New Yorkers outside HIP or similar plans are likely to be very different from those of HIP members. Willingness to use a service such as mammography, the reasons for seeking such a service, the ability to obtain an appointment, and the speed required to begin treatment when necessary may make more difference in the well-being of an individual than the technical effectiveness of the test itself. The "laboratory conditions" of the HIP investigation meant that these factors could not be studied.

Although the SLACS suffers from its own limitations (it covers only a few forms of cancer, for example), it examines early detection *in the community*. This research setting enabled the investigators to view early detection as a complex of technical capabilities and human actions. They were therefore able to examine different aspects of the early-detection process, identifying approaches that seemed especially effective and providing a perspective on the general value of early detection.

DIMENSIONS OF THE
EARLY-DETECTION PROCESS

The SLACS focused on four dimensions of the early-detection process.

The first dimension, *time from first suspicion of illness to diagnosis,* is undoubtedly the most familiar. Most people become suspicious of serious illness when they notice a symptom. The American Cancer Society and other agencies concerned with early detection have expended considerable effort in educating the public about signs possibly indicating cancer. The benefit of prompt response to a first suspicion of illness is presumably an increased chance that, should cancer actually be diagnosed, treatment may begin while the cancer is still localized and hence more likely to be cured.

A prompt response to first suspicion of illness places great responsibility on the individual. An understandable human response to the possibility of disease is to deny that a symptom exists or to hope that it will spontaneously disappear. But forces outside the individual may also influence delay. It is known, for example, that the need to pay for medical care may cause individuals to delay even when they suspect they are seriously ill.[22]

The SLACS assessed promptness of individual response to symptoms through a series of interview questions and examination of medical records. In the interviews, the researchers asked patients when they first suspected they had the illness that later proved to be cancer. Then the researchers determined from the medical record the date on which the cancer diagnosis was made. The time between these two dates was calculated in months or fractions thereof.

The second dimension studied by the SLACS was *detection at a routine physical examination.* This mechanism of early detection is essentially different from the prompt response to a cancer warning sign. It depends on observation of signs and symptoms not by the patient but by a physician during an office visit. Some observers make strong arguments for the value of early detection through routine physicals. Malignant diseases detected in this manner, it may be argued, are especially unlikely to have spread beyond their area of origin. Presumably, highly localized disease is less likely to produce perceptible symptoms than more advanced disease. A disease detected before it has developed sufficiently to alert the patient to its presence through symptoms would appear to be more readily curable. A well-known study bears out this supposition. In this study, researchers found that women with breast cancer whose malignancies were detected in routine physicians' examinations had a higher proportion of localized tumors than those who detected their own tumors accidentally and responded by seeking medical attention.[23]

In one sense, detection of cancer in a routine examination places less direct responsibility on the patient. In making an appointment for a routine examination, the individual does not face the task of directly confronting a stimulus that arouses considerable fear, as is often the case in making an appointment to have a symptom evaluated. But detection in this manner requires the patient to seek medical services in the absence of visible need, perhaps as a feature of a lifestyle emphasizing individual responsibility for health. Individual initiative, then, still plays an important role in this form of early detection.

A series of items on the SLACS questionnaire was aimed at tracing the process of cancer detection for each subject. When an individual did not identify a symptom or other cause for suspicion, the investigators inquired about how the disease was found. About one-third of the subjects indicated that their cancers were found during routine physical examinations. The term *routine physical examination* is used here in a broad, colloquial sense—synonymously with *checkup*—to encompass not only the physician's hands-on examination but other procedures associated with the encounter, including X rays, laboratory tests, etc.

The third dimension considered was *absence of pain at time of detection*. The absence of pain at the time cancer was diagnosed appeared to be an indication of early detection, resembling in some important ways the indicator just discussed, detection in a routine physical examination. In this study, patients who indicated that they had suspected cancer before obtaining a definitive diagnosis frequently became suspicious because of pain.

Seeking medical care in response to pain is not a strong indication of personal responsibility or initiative in early detection of cancer. Many who saw their physicians did so with the aim of obtaining relief from physical discomfort that they attributed to benign conditions. Several patients later found to have lung or prostate cancer, for example, had sought treatment for pain that they thought was caused by sprains or back conditions.

The fourth dimension, *prompt movement from diagnosis to treatment,* is not strictly an issue in early detection but is a crucial link between process and outcome. Examination of this aspect of the cancer patient's care acknowledges the possibility that advantages gained through early detection may be lost because of delay in treatment. Movement from diagnosis to treatment is typically outside the patient's control. Cancers are diagnosed and treated by physicians in many different specialties. The promptness with which treatment takes place depends on the availability of the appropriate specialist and the necessary facilities. The speed with which the original physician makes the referral is also a factor. Tumor registry records contain the dates at which diagnosis was made and the first course of treatment begun. This information enabled the SLACS researchers to calculate in months the time elapsed between diagnosis and the beginning of treatment.

OUTCOMES OF EARLY-DETECTION EFFORTS

These specific processes of early detection have different effects on outcomes of major interest, stage at diagnosis and survival. Table 2 indicates the relationships of two forms of the early-detection process to stage at diagnosis. According to this table, a prompt response to the symptoms has limited benefit in ensuring early-stage diagnosis for the three cancers studied. Among patients with lung cancer, those diagnosed less than two months after first suspecting they were seriously ill were found to have early-stage (Stage I) malignancies 24.5 percent of the time. This figure compares with 18.8 percent of those who waited two months or more. Among patients with cervical cancer, those who obtained diagnoses within two months had Stage I cancer 71.9 percent of the time. Those who waited two months or more had Stage I cancer 61.1 percent of the time. These small differences could well have been observed by chance. Patients with cancer of the prostate had a *poorer* chance of diagnosis in Stage I if they were diagnosed within two months of first suspecting they were seriously ill.

Table 2, however, indicates a consistent relationship between detection at a routine physical examination and early-stage diagnosis. On average, people whose cancers were detected at routine physicals were 50 percent more likely to be diagnosed in Stage I than those whose cancers were diagnosed under other circumstances—such as visits to physicians in response to symptoms. All differences were large enough so that they were probably not observed by chance.

These observations hold up under a much more detailed analysis. As statistical findings presented in Appendix B indicate, it is unlikely that the age or sex of individual patients might somehow explain the differ-

Table 2 *Early-Detection Variables and Cancer Stage*

Prompt diagnosis after first suspicion of cancer does not predict early stage.

	Percentage Early Stage	
	Suspicion to diagnosis less than two months	*Suspicion to diagnosis two months or more*
All sites	38.5	39.8
Lung	24.5	18.8
Prostate	50.3	54.8
Cervix	71.9	61.1

No differences statistically significant

Detection at a routine examination generally does predict early stage.

	Percentage Early Stage	
	Detection at routine examination	*Detection outside routine examination*
All sites	54.2	32.0
Lung	36.8	18.8
Prostate	62.3	45.5
Cervix	88.9	56.2

All differences significant ($p < .05$)

ences in stage at diagnosis shown in Table 2. This detailed analysis produced some interesting results in addition. In all three cancers, patients who had no pain at the time their diseases were detected also tended to have early-stage diagnoses. In two of the three diseases (prostate and cervix), the differences probably could not have been attributed to chance.

Prompt treatment of a patient diagnosed with cancer is an important detection-related process carried out by the health care system. But in the SLACS, this process did not seem to affect stage at diagnosis. Only a weak relationship of stage to time elapsed from diagnosis to treatment was found. All the statistics computed in this part of the analysis could well have arisen purely through chance.

With respect to the cancers studied, a clear picture emerges from these observations. Medical procedures that allow cancer to be detected *in the absence of symptoms* show strong signs of being effective. All the cancers studied are more likely to be found at an early stage if they are discovered at a routine physical examination. In two of the three cancers, the absence of pain at the time the disease was detected predicted early-stage diagnosis. A prompt diagnosis following first suspicion of illness (because of the presence of symptoms) had a much weaker relation to early-stage diagnosis. Among the malignancies studied here, the relationship was statistically significant only for cervical cancer.

The key question in early detection is, of course, "Do the patients survive?" Each of the early-detection mechanisms examined here is an aspect of the process of cancer detection, and survival is the final outcome. Figure 6 illustrates the relationships between early-detection mechanisms and five-year survival. The findings presented in this figure are not directly observed percentages; instead, they are estimates based on a statistical model that determines the effects of various early-detection methods on five-year survival after important background characteristics (such as age and sex) have been taken into account.

Consistent with the relationships between early-detection mechanisms and early-stage diagnosis of cancer, Figure 6 suggests only a limited role for prompt diagnosis following first suspicion of illness. When lung, prostatic, and cervical cancers are combined, delay of less than two months corresponds to an increase in five-year survival that is too small to rule out having been observed by chance. Only women with cervical cancer obtain a statistically significant survival advantage.

Figure 6, however, strongly suggests that detection of cancer at a routine physical effectively promotes five-year survival. When all cancer patients are examined as a single group, those who had their cancers detected at a routine physical clearly evidenced a greater likelihood of surviving five years than those who did not. This relationship is true, moreover, of all the cancers studied. The survival differences between those who had their diseases detected at a routine physical and those who did not are large enough to rule out chance observation in all three cancers.

It is important to remember, as discussed earlier in this book, that five-year survival is not always the best way to assess the cure or control of a malignancy. For this reason, the SLACS researchers compared the

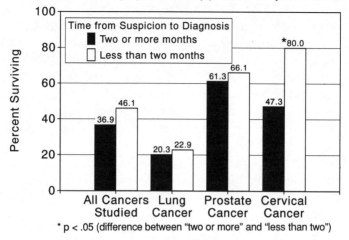

Prompt response to symptoms weakly predicts five-year survival.

* p < .05 (difference between "two or more" and "less than two")

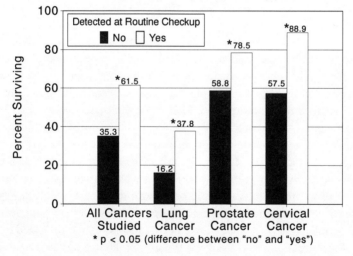

But detection at a routine checkup is a strong predictor.

* p < 0.05 (difference between "no" and "yes")

Fig. 6. *Early detection and five-year survival rates.*

risks of death over the course of the study for different groups (relative mortality risks). Like the statistical model associated with Figure 6, estimation of relative mortality risk took account of age, sex, and cancer site—all potentially important factors in treatment and survival. This analysis indicated that prompt diagnosis following suspicion of illness reduced mortality risk only for cervical cancer. But diagnosis at a routine physical examination reduced mortality risk for all three cancers. The reduction in risk is greater than attributable to chance in analyses combining all three cancers and in separate analyses of lung and prostatic cancer.

The researchers also assessed the effects of cancer detection in the absence of pain. Highly similar findings emerged. People without pain had more favorable rates of five-year survival and a decreased relative mortality risk.

Are the Survival Advantages Real?

Before interpreting these observations or applying the lessons learned, we need to ask some basic questions about what the numbers cited above actually mean. Biomedical scientists have questioned whether data suggesting that early detection prolongs survival have been correctly interpreted. They point out that a statistical problem known as the "zero time shift" or "lead-time bias" may make the lives of people whose cancers were identified through early detection seem longer—but that the increased life expectancy is a mirage. According to an authoritative source, "This phenomenon occurs when a screening test or other appropriate diagnostic procedure leads to the detection of a disease before symptoms have developed. Even if therapy is ineffectual, the period of survival will be increased by the increment provided by the presymptomatic detection of the disease."[24] That is to say, researchers may err in considering that patients have a survival advantage when cancer is detected and treated before warning signs appear. Those who have their diseases diagnosed and treated may not benefit from starting treatment earlier in the natural history of their disease. In reality, they may only be acknowledged earlier as having cancer and observed longer between diagnosis and death than those diagnosed after the appearance of symptoms.

According to statistics computed in the SLACS, patients diagnosed while free of symptoms—indicated by the absence of pain (the most frequently reported symptom) or the detection of cancer at a routine physical—had better chances of five-year survival and a lower relative risk. Did these patients really live longer? Were they "cured" more often? Or did the tumor registry merely acknowledge their illness at an earlier point in its natural history, at which time it was no more likely to be cured than if it had progressed far enough to produce symptoms?

To resolve this dilemma, the SLACS investigators reasoned that a closer examination of the disease process was necessary. Stage is perhaps the most important marker in the disease process, reflecting the degree of dissemination of the malignancy. If diagnosis at an earlier stage could be established as the *mechanism* of life extension in those whose cancers were detected in the absence of symptoms, there would be less possibility that these individuals were merely observed longer and not cured more frequently. The investigators sought evidence that early detection resulted in diagnosis at an early stage and that this early diagnosis resulted in the extension of life. If no such evidence would be found, they reasoned, extension of life would be illusory.

Consistent with this perspective, the researchers analyzed the relationships between early detection and survival, to see whether these relationships remained after any possible impact of stage as an intermediate step was removed. If the relationships between early detection and survival remained, they postulated, stage could not have served as the operative mechanism; and such a finding would strengthen the possibility that longer survival was recorded merely because patients were followed longer.

The connection between early detection and survival typically became much weaker when the influence of stage was eliminated. Five-year survival in prostate and cervical cancer provides the most straightforward illustration. In Figure 6, where the influence of stage was not controlled, statistically significant relations between detection at a routine physical and five-year survival were visible for all the diseases studied. When stage is held constant, however, the relationship is no longer significant for either prostate or cervical cancer. Relationships between absence of pain at diagnosis and five-year survival become weaker as well when stage is held constant. A similar pattern occurs in analysis of relative mortality risk.

Lung cancer proved to be more complex. The relation between detection at a routine physical and survival remained after stage was held constant in an analysis including all the lung cancer patients interviewed.

But analysis of the subgroup most likely to respond well to curative treatment produced results similar to those found for prostatic and cervical cancer. This subgroup (about 40 percent of all the lung cancer patients interviewed) included patients sixty-five years of age and under, diagnosed at Stage I or II, and having only non–small cell disease. Within this subgroup, the strength of the relationship between detection at a routine physical and relative mortality risk fell by about 20 percent and was no longer statistically significant after the effect of stage was controlled.

In view of these findings, it seems unlikely that the effects of early detection reported here reflect mere statistical bias. Direct observation indicates a relationship between early detection (either at a routine physical or in the absence of pain) and early-stage diagnosis. Stage itself appears to provide the linkage between early detection and enhanced survival.

◆   ◆   ◆   ◆   ◆

Generally, the widely shared belief in the benefits of early detection appears to be no myth. *Early detection has a real and meaningful effect on survival.* For the majority of patients in the SLACS investigation, at least some early-detection mechanisms appeared effective in enhancing survival. The reservations of some concerning the applicability of this approach to improving cancer survival seem to be exaggerated.

But the approach to early detection that seems most promising in the cancers studied here differs from the approach that has traditionally received the widest publicity. The processes that seem most effective do *not* rely on the individual's reaction to symptoms. They take place, in fact, when the cancer is detected in the absence of early signals. This is not to say that we as individuals may abdicate responsibility for cancer survival in our personal lives. Everyone should still see a physician as soon as possible in response to a cancer warning signal. For some cancers not studied here, the benefits of prompt response to symptoms are almost certainly greater. But for cancer in general, the most important personal responsibility may be to obtain routine physical examinations. For many individuals, however, factors over which they have little personal control—including income, education, and the availability of medical resources—may make this responsibility virtually impossible to exercise. The following chapter will explore the impacts of these factors.

Before we consider such questions, further issues need to be raised about the specialized system that carries out cancer-related medical services. Details of the patient interviews suggest that researchers should pay increased attention to delay within the diagnostic process itself. While patients are not "expert" reporters, their stories suggest that cancer diagnosis in community settings may involve significant miscommunication and error. These stories remind us that diagnosis can be technically complex. Cancers themselves may be masked by other conditions. Physicians are not always attentive to cancer signs. Several cases illustrate these problems.

A fifty-five-year-old woman, later found to have Stage II lung cancer, complained to her physician of fatigue, coughing, and a chronic sore throat. Her physician diagnosed the condition as bronchitis and prescribed medications. The condition initially improved, but recurred in six months. The physician again treated her for bronchitis, and her condition improved. This process was repeated several more times, until the patient began spitting up blood and was seen in an emergency room. Another physician eventually made the correct diagnosis.

A seventy-year-old man developed a very bad cough while away on vacation. After returning home, he saw his physician, but no disease was found. He returned for tests including X rays, bronchoscopies, and a biopsy. Many were negative. After more than seven months of this testing, a positive diagnosis of Stage II lung cancer was made. The man died ten months after diagnosis.

A patient diagnosed with Stage II prostatic cancer reported seeing his physician because of pain and difficulty in eating. He returned to this physician several times over a nine-month period, but was told that he was "fine" and that he only had pain, which could not be treated. The patient felt that his physician was not attentive to his symptoms. Finally, he went to a new physician, who made the diagnosis. A seventy-three-year-old man, this patient died about three years after his diagnosis.

A sixty-six-year-old patient saw her physician for swelling in the head and neck. The doctor diagnosed the condition as mumps. When the condition did not improve after a week, the physician ordered X rays, which indicated a tumor. The patient was diagnosed with Stage II lung cancer and died about five months later.

A fifty-five-year-old patient saw his physician for a pain in his shoulder. He was initially given muscle relaxants, which brought partial relief. The patient died five months after the subsequent diagnosis of lung cancer.

Suspecting a serious problem, a sixty-eight-year-old man visited a physician for a pain in his groin. The physician diagnosed the condition as a hernia. About two years elapsed between the man's initial suspicion and the ultimate diagnosis of Stage I prostate cancer. Six years after his diagnosis, however, the man remained alive.

These patient interviews do not constitute hard data. The people who died might not have survived appreciably longer if their diagnoses had been swifter and surer. The nature of some cases makes the diagnostic process difficult for the most skilled physician. Nonetheless, leaders of the medical profession and individual physicians should acknowledge the importance of cancer-detection skills. The findings presented in this chapter support the notion that every doctor's office should be a cancer-detection center, as the American Cancer Society has urged. If they are to play this role, health professionals must possess adequate cancer-detection skills, pay sufficient attention to patient complaints, and communicate complex and fear-arousing information effectively. As consumers, patients have responsibility for selecting physicians who possess these capabilities.

CHAPTER SEVEN

Class and Cancer Survival

Class, an individual's standing in society's hierarchy of resources, esteem, and power over others, affects most aspects of life—including, perhaps especially, health and longevity. This chapter examines the influence of class on the cancer patient's chances for survival. Consideration of class continues this book's focus on factors in cancer survival outside the traditional concerns of biology and medicine. An examination of class has particular importance in identifying forces that simultaneously affect the outlook and behavior of large numbers of individuals, and thus the survival chances of millions of cancer patients.

Chapters 5 and 6 examined factors in cancer survival more closely related to the individual patient's thinking and behavior than medical research or treatment. Chapter 5 provided no evidence that a person's emotional state affects his or her chance of survival. But, according to Chapter 6, the individual's habits regarding medical care seem to be significant. People who saw a physician on a routine basis, whether or not they had symptoms, greatly increased their chances for early diagnosis and survival. Those who saw their physicians *in response to* symptoms sometimes improved their survival chances, but not as consistently as those who took prospective action. The technical efficacy of early-detection methods available in the late twentieth century was a crucial factor in cancer survival for many. But the individual's outlook and decisions regarding utilization of this technology appeared crucial as well.

This and the next chapter shift attention from individual to social factors, which affect willingness and ability to obtain health care. Both the resources commanded by people as individuals and features of the health care system itself participate in this process. They encourage people to seek care or deter them from seeking it, and they influence people's choice of providers—which, in turn, may affect quality of care.

Nonbiomedical factors in cancer survival go well beyond the thinking and habits of individuals. Powerful forces in the world around them influence the behavior and outlook of men and women. The level of encouragement they receive for taking action on their own behalf has much to do with determining the length and quality of their lives, whether or not they develop cancer or another serious illness. The organization of health care—briefly, the manner in which health care professionals are coordinated, motivated, and paid—strongly influences the individual's ability to obtain appropriate care in time for it to be most effective. A large part of the action taken by individuals stems from conditions of their lives, and reflects the quality of life in the society of which they are part.

This chapter focuses on the individual's resources; the next chapter focuses on a key development in the organization of the health care system. Changes in the system appear likely to affect patients in different ways, depending on their health problems and resources. These changes will affect cancer survival, no matter what treatments and cures scientists and physicians may develop in the coming century. Americans must acknowledge that class membership strongly influences the health care people seek and receive, and they must assess the changes now occurring with this fact in mind.

Class and Health Care

Class is America's "dirty little secret." We take pride that our civilization has offered opportunity to so many. We do our best to ignore distinctions of wealth and schooling. The stockbroker jokes with the shoeshine boy; the politician, no matter how patrician his lineage, strives to use the language of the common man. But the human pecking order manifests its importance at the true turning points of life. Understanding the relationship between the individual's position in the social order and his or her chances for surviving serious illness helps illustrate this principle—and has major implications for our personal lives and direction as a community.

The 1960s brought a public commitment to equality, with programs such as Medicare and Medicaid giving the elderly and the poor access to America's vast health care resources. But in the late twentieth century, equality did not materialize. At least on the visual level, the places where rich and poor people go for health care contrast markedly. A visit to a ghetto health clinic would jar middle-class sensibilities. Waiting rooms are full. Amenities are scarce. Children are numerous and noisy. The lady at the front desk looks puzzled when handed a card from a private insurance plan or offered cash; her experience is almost entirely with Medicaid clients. When they are called, usually after a long wait, patients may see a physician assistant, nurse practitioner, or other "physician extender" instead of the doctor. Because Medicaid payments are well below what physicians are accustomed to receiving, those who accept Medicaid patients often turn to high-volume practice, shortening encounters with patients to a minimum and delegating work to aides whenever possible. Such "Medicaid mills" may dominate health care in the disadvantaged community.

The county hospital, which mainly serves poor people, may be even more shocking to middle-class eyes. Corridors in the clinic areas and around the emergency room are crowded. The atmosphere is odorous. Fixtures and equipment are old. People waiting to be seen for everyday complaints may share the facility with derelicts from the street, rowdies injured in fights, inmates brought under guard from the county jail. Waiting is prolonged as ambulances deliver trauma victims. Behind the scenes, physicians-in-training tremble as they face their first assignments in suturing. Underpaid nurses express exasperation. An overworked supervising physician struggles to exercise adequate oversight.

Health care for the super rich might just as well be delivered on a different planet. John D. Rockefeller, history's best-known tycoon, is said to have maintained fully equipped hospitals for his private use in the basements of his many mansions. Today's elites may enjoy health care in settings only slightly less sumptuous. On a floor called the "Gold Coast," a Los Angeles hospital caters exclusively to the special needs of the privileged. The floors are richly carpeted. Original art adorns the walls. Small rooms adjoin those of the patients, allowing maids and valets to remain close at hand. On a recent stay, a famous actress brought her own silverware and dishes. A prominent "community leader" brought his bodyguards. For the international set, a hospital in London maintains a staff of five-star chefs and a world-class wine cellar. One can only guess at the settings in which the presidents and dictators of the modern world receive their medical care.

In view of these almost unbelievable differences, it is impossible to ignore the fundamental question: Do the elite have a better chance of surviving life-threatening diseases such as cancer? Physicians differ in their opinions. Some maintain that the differences between the county hospital and the Gold Coast are superficial. As far as actual medical care is concerned, it is argued, the rich enjoy no material advantage. The same physician may see both rich and poor patients, dividing his or her time between facilities serving the rich and the poor—the former to generate income, the latter to take advantage of research opportunities and perform community service.

Other physicians disagree. True, the individual practitioner may attempt to serve both the upper and lower classes, but the number of physicians who maintain steady commitments in both areas is unknown. Even skilled, committed physicians seem to experience difficulty providing quality service in settings specializing in care for the poor. They report shortages of supplies. They note that the skills of support personnel may be weak. They tell stories of lost records and X rays. The high volume of patients may strain concentration and communication. Frequent turnover of health professionals may create problems in coordinating early and later phases of treatment.

By the late twentieth century, the worlds of rich and poor were further apart than they had been at the close of the 1960s. As described in Chapter 1, public commitments to equality in health care declined as the years wore on and costs increased. In the 1960s, it had been expected that Medicaid would empty the big city and county hospitals whose clinics had served as the sole sources of care for the poor. But by the 1980s, the fees Medicaid paid to physicians had shrunk to the point where many no longer accepted Medicaid patients in their practices. New regulations in many jurisdictions mandated that hospitals compete for contracts to serve Medicaid patients, submitting bids to state governments that administered the program. The poor were willingly received only at hospitals that had won the competition—in part by offering low-priced services. State regulations made it harder to qualify for Medicaid, removing thousands of "working poor" from the rolls. These, and the transient, the alien, and the homeless, turned up at the county hospitals as they always had. At other facilities, administrative personnel made sure that those who could not pay were directed elsewhere.

The contrast between the settings in which rich and poor receive services is striking. But this comparison merely sets the stage for problems shared by the broad spectrum of Americans. Rich and poor people comprise only a small percentage of the American public. Most of us are middle class—and face increasing difficulties in obtaining services to which we feel entitled.

The American middle class still enjoys a standard of living envied throughout the world. Except in recessions and during runs of bad luck, middle-class people have steady jobs, which usually provide health insurance as a fringe benefit. Prudent workers save for health emergencies. Steady income and health insurance allow middle-class people to see private doctors on a regular basis, in much more appealing settings than those facing the poor. Middle-class people have always enjoyed significant choice over the physicians they see. Savings may allow them to seek out potentially effective treatments not covered by their insurance. For the middle-class elderly, savings and pension income supplement Medicare sufficiently to ensure access to the same health care that was available to them while they were still working.

But the late twentieth century brought changes in health care that weakened these advantages. The costs of health care grew at an unbelievable rate. Even the steadily employed began to see their personal outlays for health care rising. As late as the 1970s, many employers provided first-dollar coverage for health care to their employees; the employee paid nothing, no matter how much health care he or she required. But by the 1990s, almost all employee health plans included deductibles and copayments. Deductibles require the employee to pay a stipulated amount of the medical bill before insurance becomes effective; copayments require the employee to cover a percentage of each bill even after the deductible. It was not uncommon to find workers who paid thousands of dollars for themselves and their family members before their insurance kicked in. The 20 percent typically required for copayments—this requirement became standard in both employee insurance plans and Medicare—could amount to a substantial sum. A "golden age" of health insurance had given way to an era when the middle class again had to make substantial health care payments out of pocket.

The weakening of benefits relied on for so long by the middle class underscores the importance of the relationship between position in the social order and survival of serious illness. Personal resources become more important as the social safety net unravels. The middle class is not immune. While America's living standard may still engender envy from the rest of the world, its system of financing health care provokes fear abroad. Foreign governments and travel agents warn voyagers bound for the United States that a health emergency will be treated very differently than in their native land. Should they need health care in the United States, they will have to pay for it—and more than they ever dreamed possible!

This chapter asks how a person's place on the totem pole affects his or her chance of surviving cancer. Americans believe in equality. But everyone knows that people occupy different stations in life. Americans don't talk much about class. But we see class distinctions every day in the neighborhoods we live in, the cars we drive, the schools our children attend. Class distinctions—"social stratification," the sociologist or anthropologist might say—are a fact of life.

Information about the effects that class may have on cancer survival is vital for several reasons. A good society, many believe, should see to it that survival of cancer or other serious diseases does not depend on position in the social order. If the disease can be controlled for some, it should be controlled for all. The existence of class differences in survival should forcefully remind us of how far we have strayed from the ideal of equality in health care. Since such a morally distinguished— though perhaps economically unfeasible—position probably will not be adopted, an understanding of the relationship between social class and survival may at least lay a groundwork for programs specifically targeted at reducing preventable cancer mortality among the disadvantaged.

More important to people as individuals, an understanding of the relationship between class and cancer survival can provide guidelines for personal action. Personal resources create opportunities for the individual to raise his or her chances for surviving cancer. Not everyone takes full advantage of these opportunities. The obituaries of the rich regularly report deaths from cancers of types that are often diagnosed early and treated successfully. Determining the mechanisms by which social and economic advantages result in better survival chances suggests ways in which individuals with these resources—or the inventiveness to compensate for resources they lack—may make the most of them.

Definitions of Class

The concept of class is extremely powerful. Through the ages, it has instigated social movements, civil unrest, wars, revolutions, and purges. Many thinkers regard classes as communities of individuals who share common levels of control over the economy and political institutions—the U.S. Congress, state legislatures, the Republican and Democratic parties. Karl Marx is the most famous proponent of this view. Under such a notion of class, people who share similar levels of wealth and power constitute a group that realizes its shared interests and directs the political machinery of the state to safeguard them. In this sense, class functions at a level well above and removed from the day-to-day fortunes of individuals. Class is seen as an instrument of great historical transformations, not as a mere measure of personal resources.

Class has played an important and visible role in the history of modern Europe. European political parties with names like "labor" and "socialist" nurture and draw support from class sympathies. Such class consciousness has not occurred with permanence or regularity in America. Historically, too many other things have been going on. Coming from every corner of the earth, immigrants to the United States tended to identify more closely with their ethnicity than with their class position. Race has played a much more important part in American public life than class has. To many Americans, the real divisions in society are not rich versus poor but black versus white. Finally, the frontier spirit has distracted Americans from cares about social divisions. In the 1800s, a person who was unhappy with his or her position in society could find a new life in the West. Although the frontier may have ceased to exist in the 1890s, it survived in American culture through the twentieth century. Generations of Americans have been trained to think of their individual capabilities and achievements—not class solidarity or social revolution—as the most important determinants of success and happiness.

Consistent with this history and culture, American social scientists tend to view class as an array of distinct resources and characteristics that an individual may possess, rather than as a coherent identity. These resources may include material assets, such as income, and less tangible attributes, such as prestige. An individual's class position in this sense is still important, even though it does not necessarily involve questions of social change.

Variables such as income, education, and prestige reflect the overall "life chances" of the individual.[1] Even in a society like the United States, which offers significant opportunity for individual achievement, class thought of in this way is important. The class into which one is born will have much to do with how much money he or she earns and how much deference, respect, honor, and obedience he or she receives from others.[2] Moving upward through the class structure allows the individual not just to consume more expensive goods and services but to associate and communicate with a broader range of people.[3]

The social scientist in modern America thinks of class in terms closely associated with the activities of everyday life. The modern social scientist, in fact, hesitates to use the word *class,* preferring instead terms such as *social status* or *stratum.* These words suggest that society, like a layer cake or rock formation, is divided into a stable set of levels. People who find themselves in one layer may envy those in the layers above and move upward themselves—this is "social mobility." But the hallmark of the ordering is that it itself is stable. The members of one stratum do not band together to fight a class war and seize power from another. Unlike the Marxists of yesteryear, modern social scientists tend to view the social order as an arrangement of categories of people with differing levels of access to goods and services.

But consumption of goods and services does not tell the whole story. Class has an important subjective dimension as well. While social stratum does not define sides in a class war, it seems to help determine self-perception, lifestyle, and culture.[4] Americans do not like to think of themselves as members of classes in conflict with each other, but they seem aware that they occupy different levels in society. A strong degree of consensus exists among Americans about which jobs command the most respect.[5] The individual's level in this hierarchy helps determine his or her self-confidence and range of social contacts. A mechanic interviewed in a classic study, for example, distinguished himself within the pecking order as a person who *handled* tasks rather than planned them for others. This distinction spilled over into social contacts: " '[The man who plans work for others] doesn't feel out of place when he's associating with men like professors, lawyers, and doctors—and oh say—bankers. He doesn't feel that he's out of place. He associates with them and he's sure of himself.' "[6]

People who perceive themselves as working class do not necessarily feel inferior to those who wear white collars and neckties to their jobs.

Each stratum seems to have its own code of honor. People who "handle" things often express a sense of pride in knowing that the higher-ups depend on them. George Meany, the national labor leader who began in the plumbers' union, once remarked that a city could get along very well without lawyers but would run into trouble rapidly without members of his own trade. Strata not ordinarily considered dominant on the national level have historically taken care of tasks on which the country depends, and they consider this role a source of pride from generation to generation. The professional military is a key example.[7]

Although American citizens and social scientists alike shy away from the rhetoric of class, then, both seem aware of major divisions within the social order. These social divisions seem to break along the lines of visible resources and attributes of individuals—income, education, and occupational prestige. Even in the United States, with its strong belief in equality, position in the social order—call it status, class, stratum, or some other term—is a major determinant in the course of our lives. It plays a large part in determining our habits and beliefs, our choice of marriage partners, our success in the world of work, and our lives as retired people. It is natural that class should affect our health care, our health itself, and our ability to survive and recover in the event of cancer and other serious diseases.

For purposes of convenience, the following discussion uses terms such as *class, social stratum,* and *socioeconomic status* interchangeably. Each of these terms is simply intended to denote the position of the individual in the social and economic hierarchy. The United States is a country where individual dimensions of this ordering—wealth, education, prestige—need not coalesce in the same individual. The following discussion distinguishes among these dimensions only when necessary to attain a sharper understanding of who survives cancer.

Social Class and Mortality Risk

Generations of researchers have studied the relationship between class, health, and survival. They have uncovered consistent evidence that the lower an individual's position on the socioeconomic-status ladder, the greater his or her chance of contracting serious illness and the shorter his or her life expectancy. In centuries past, the fabled excesses of the gentry may have predisposed them to certain diseases, a fatty diet and freedom from physical labor easing them into the "gout syndrome" as they matured. The better access to medical care these advantaged people may have enjoyed probably did them more harm than good. But when the entire life cycle is considered, the privileged almost certainly enjoyed an overall advantage. The impact of class on illness, health, and survival has certainly been apparent since the industrial revolution. Its continuation even in the modern welfare state is especially baffling and disturbing.

Living conditions in eighteenth- and nineteenth-century Europe and America, and in the Third World today, translate economic disadvantages into health risks. In societies where a large segment of the population lacks basic nutrition, permanent housing, potable water, and sewers, the poorest often die of diseases directly related to their poverty. Lacking access to a safe water supply, for example, today's Third World poor face significant risks of death from infantile diarrhea, cholera, and typhoid. Wealthier people rarely encounter such risks.

In the United States and other industrial countries, even the poorest usually drink from safe water supplies, have access to public nutrition programs, and qualify for basic health services at public clinics and hospitals. Massive epidemics of infectious diseases, which selectively attacked the poor and socially disadvantaged, ceased after the introduction of immunization in the early and mid-twentieth century. It is surprising, then, to see that distinctions in health and longevity between the relatively more and less advantaged persisted through the century, even in the rich, industrialized countries of Europe and America.

In the United States, socioeconomic status has long had an impact on life expectancy. A landmark study by sociologists Evelyn Kitagawa and Philip Hauser provides an illustration.[8] These researchers examined life expectancy in Chicago between 1930 and 1960. In that period, average life span increased within all social groupings. Life expectancy increased faster for nonwhites than for whites. Still, by the end of the study period, whites continued to live longer on the average. But upon detailed analysis, longevity proved to depend more on class than on race. Differences between nonwhites and whites disappeared when membership in the lower classes, which tended to characterize nonwhites, was taken into account.

Even in Great Britain, with its strong welfare state and a National Health Service providing care for all citizens at public expense, higher socioeconomic status generally means a longer life. Unsure about the effectiveness of the National Health Service in eliminating inequalities of class, the British secretary of state for social services appointed a commission headed by Sir Douglas Black, president of the Royal College of Physicians, to assess differences in mortality between the upper and lower strata and recommend how these differences could be reduced. The product of this commission is known as the Black Report, and is read by public health officials throughout the world.[9] Living in a country where some people still have titles of nobility and a monarch still reigns, English people seem much more willing than Americans to use the word *class* and to confront class distinctions.

To assess the effects of class on longevity, Sir Douglas's group chose a scale based on occupation as a convenient though inexact method of identifying an individual's class. They reasoned that occupation determines not only family income but conditions of work and associated health risks as well. The categories included in the scale, and the percentage of "economically active" and retired people in each of them during the early 1970s, are as follows:

    I. *Professional* (for example, accountant, doctor, lawyer): 5 percent
   II. *Intermediate* (manager, nurse, teacher, etc.): 18 percent
IIIN. *Skilled Nonmanual* (clerical worker, secretary): 12 percent
IIIM. *Skilled Manual* (bus driver, carpenter, butcher): 38 percent
  IV. *Partly Skilled* (agricultural worker, postman): 18 percent
   V. *Unskilled* (laborer): 9 percent

When deaths occur in England, the Registrar General's office routinely records the decedent's own occupation and that of his or her next of kin according to this set of categories. For nonworking wives and children, the husband's occupation is taken as the class indicator. Division of the number of deaths within a given class by the total number of individuals in that class, a figure obtainable from the census, yields the mortality rate for each class, making comparisons possible.

Using records assembled in the early 1970s, the researchers found that persons in Class V were 2.5 times more likely to die before retirement than those in Class I, even when age differences were statistically controlled. Perhaps most interesting was the observation that mortality risk tended to increase steadily from Class I through Class V. Thus, a skilled manual worker (or his or her spouse or child) had a higher risk of dying than a lawyer or teacher. Persons in the "skilled manual" and "professional" classes did not differ in their ability to obtain necessities such as food and shelter, but they did differ in mortality risk. The Black Report documented this "mortality gradient" for accidents and nearly all infectious and noninfectious diseases, including heart disease and cancer.

The class distinction in death rates is especially striking in Great Britain, which, by the 1970s, had had health care provided without charge to all citizens for close to forty years. The researchers explained their findings in several ways. Lifestyle appeared to play a role, with people in lower-level occupations more often being smokers and less often consuming a healthy diet. But those with lower-level occupations also used health services (general practitioner physicians and hospitals) less often, even when the comparison was adjusted for medical need.

A review of mortality records going back to the 1920s outlined a similar picture—namely, that people in lower-level occupations faced higher mortality risks. The years between 1949 and 1972 were especially important. Throughout this period, England received its health care from the National Health Service. In these years, mortality risk decreased among the young and the upper social classes. But for older members of the lower classes, death rates remained the same or, for some groups, increased. Overall, social-class differences in mortality risk became larger.[10]

An important study in Canada revealed similar findings. In 1971, an individual's income provided a good clue to his or her mortality risks.[11] Researchers in this study compared five different income categories. Their statistics indicate that, in nearly every age group, people in lower-income categories had higher risks of dying. The difference was observed even when comparisons were made for specific diseases, such as heart disease or cancer. This study is especially important for the United States. In the early 1970s, Canada's health care system was very much like our own, with people seeing private doctors and usually paying through private insurance. Furthermore, seemingly small income differences made important differences in mortality risk. People whose incomes differed by as little as $2,000 had different life expectancies.

Major studies have indicated that, all in all, people lower in the social order have shorter lives and experience higher risks than those higher up. But these studies do not go very far in determining why this is so. Do the resources and lifestyles associated with higher status have this impact only by keeping people well? Or do the relatively advantaged have a better chance of recovering from life-threatening illnesses? An analysis of the relationship between major social distinctions and survival among people with cancer helps answer this question.

Social Factors and Cancer Survival in the United States

RACE AND ETHNICITY

In the United States, race and ethnicity are the most obvious places to begin an inquiry into the social and economic factors that affect an individual's chance for surviving cancer. Americans focus first and foremost on race when they deal with public issues. In the area of cancer survival, this focus is warranted. The relationship between race and cancer survival in the United States is well documented and striking.

Researchers at the National Cancer Institute have followed hundreds of thousands of people with cancer, to determine the relationships between race, ethnicity, and cancer survival. One major study compared blacks and whites from several widely separated parts of the United States who were diagnosed with cancer between 1960 and 1973.[12] Blacks who developed cancer during this period had a considerably lower probability of surviving five years than whites. Some of this difference appeared to be related to early detection. Whereas 40 percent of white patients had their diseases diagnosed while still localized, 30 percent of black patients were diagnosed at this early stage. In a total of eighteen types of cancers studied by these scientists, about 40 percent of white patients survived, compared with 30 percent of the black patients. Among patients diagnosed with Hodgkin's disease between 1967 and 1973, 61 percent of the whites survived five years or longer. For black patients, the figure was 46 percent.

Even when they were diagnosed at the same stage, black patients had poorer survival chances than white patients. For all cancers, 68 percent of the white patients diagnosed between 1967 and 1973 with early-stage disease survived five years, compared with 62 percent of blacks. In some cancers, the differences were much greater. Whites with localized lung cancer had a 34 percent five-year survival rate, compared with 22 percent for blacks. For localized cancer of the rectum and bladder, five-year survival rates for white and black patients were 69 versus 53 percent and 72 versus 53 percent.

During this period, researchers detected differences in survival rates between racial and ethnic groups other than white and black. Following patients diagnosed between 1967 and 1979, scientists at the National Cancer Institute compared survival among "Anglos," blacks, Hispanics, American Indians, Chinese, Japanese, Filipinos, and Hawaiians.[13] Survival rates for each of these groups differed for the various forms of cancer. But some groups usually enjoyed advantages, others disadvantages. Japanese generally had highly favorable five-year survival rates. In colon cancer, Japanese had a five-year survival rate of 59 percent; Anglos, 49; and blacks, 44. For prostate cancer, Japanese had a five-year survival rate of 74 percent; Anglos, 66; and blacks, 56. For women with breast cancer, five-year survival rates for these ethnic groups were 84, 73, and 61 percent. Like the blacks, American Indians and Filipinos usually had less favorable survival chances than Anglos.

Specialized studies in Hawaii, with its strong representation of many Asian ethnicities, confirmed the National Cancer Institute's findings with respect to Japanese, Chinese, Filipinos, and Caucasians.[14] In breast and lung cancers, Japanese had the best chance for five-year survival, followed by Caucasians, Chinese, and Filipinos.

SOCIOECONOMIC STATUS

Although socioeconomic status receives less public attention in the United States than race or ethnicity, the cancer patient's place in the social and economic hierarchy is clearly a harbinger of his or her survival. A number of research studies in a wide variety of settings have demonstrated the importance of socioeconomic status. While methods of inquiry and analysis vary, the findings have been quite consistent.

An early California study followed cancer patients listed in a state tumor registry between 1942 and 1962. The researchers compared patients who sought care at public hospitals with those treated in private hospitals, assuming that the private-hospital patients would be of a higher class than those in the public hospitals. At diagnosis, cancers among the private-hospital patients were early stage (localized) twice as often as those in the public hospitals. Patients treated in private hospitals were more likely to survive five years or longer for every type of malignancy studied.[15]

Two later regional studies produced similar findings. In a study based in Connecticut and Massachusetts, investigators compared patients residing in census tracts—the neighborhood-sized areas defined by the

Census Bureau for purposes of comparison—with median incomes below and above $5,000 in 1960. Patients from the poorer areas had lower short-term survival.[16] A study at the University of Iowa Hospital compared paying patients with charity patients and found that the paying, presumably more affluent, patients were more likely to survive five or more years.[17]

The sophistication of researchers has increased over the years, and some now doubt that socioeconomic status has a major effect on cancer survival after background factors such as age and disease severity have explained all they can.[18] But the more sophisticated analyses suggest that general class differences in survival, although they may be relatively weak, become strong when comparisons are made only among people with certain cancers. An Ohio researcher, for example, has reported that the strongest survival differences between lower- and higher-class people occur among those with "less severe" forms of gastrointestinal cancer— small intestine, colon, and rectum, as opposed to stomach, liver, and pancreas.[19]

The most important studies of class and cancer survival, however, are those indicating not only that class influences survival chances but also that class explains away any impact of race. Nobody disputes that some racial minorities—blacks, American Indians, and Filipinos, for example—face higher risks of mortality when they contract cancer. But a strong consensus among researchers is emerging that the lower socioeconomic status associated with membership in these minority groups explains the unfavorable odds faced by their members. Race itself is not the cause.

In one important study, researchers followed 1,032 black and 1,481 white men diagnosed with prostate cancer between 1968 and 1977.[20] Subjects were drawn from eleven comprehensive cancer centers throughout the United States that had high representations of both black and white patients. The researchers estimated the patients' socioeconomic status by the census tract in which they resided. Those who lived in areas with high rates of high school or college graduation were considered high socioeconomic status; those in areas with low graduation rates, low status. In the analysis of differences in mortality risk, blacks at first appeared at higher risk. But when socioeconomic status was held constant, the influence of race disappeared. Low socioeconomic status indicated higher mortality risk, however, even when race was controlled.

A year after the release of the prostate cancer investigation, another research team made public the results of a study comparing black and white women with breast cancer.[21] The researchers in this study followed 1,506 women for eleven years after they were diagnosed. Like most studies of socioeconomic status and mortality risk, this study assessed class on the basis of the subject's census tract. The researchers examined a wider variety of items related to class than most earlier investigators, including educational level in the census tract, percentage below 125 percent of the poverty line, and percentage of families living on public assistance. Furthermore, they designated patients as inside or outside the "working class." Those in the working class lived in areas where a high percentage of the employed people did not own businesses or employ or supervise other people. The researchers found that women in the working class had a 50 percent higher risk of dying over the course of the study than women outside the working class. When the influence of race was first examined, black women had a mortality rate one-third higher than whites. But when the effect of class was removed, black women did not differ from whites.

Acutely interested in reducing excess cancer mortality among the disadvantaged, the American Cancer Society set up a study group to examine in depth the influence of socioeconomic status on cancer survival. The group, called the Committee on Cancer in the Economically Disadvantaged, issued its final report in 1986, after a comprehensive review of all foregoing research on class, race, and other social factors related to cancer mortality. The committee acknowledged that race might reflect cultural factors, which, in turn, might have an impact on behavior related to health and the use of medical care. But the committee concluded that "ethnic differences"—the most important being those between black and white—in cancer survival are "largely secondary to socioeconomic factors and associated processes."[22]

A great deal of uncertainty, however, accompanies this consensus. Experts do not know why socially and economically disadvantaged cancer patients have lower chances for survival. Some speculate that the disadvantaged experience longer delays in cancer detection and treatment. But many investigators, reporting that high-status people have survival advantages even when stage is controlled, believe that early detection does not serve as the link between class and survival. Others suggest that the advantaged have a better survival chance because they obtain higher-quality care. An important investigation of prostate cancer patients at the Veterans Administration found no racial differences in survival; the authors suggest that equality of health care, which would prevail among VA patients, reduces the disadvantages in survival that racial minorities might otherwise face.[23] But equal quality of services should also have prevailed in the University of Iowa study, where all patients were presumably seen in the same clinics. Nonindigent patients were still more likely to survive than indigent patients.

To improve individual survival chances and reduce the disadvantages faced by those lower in the social order, individuals and policymakers need more information about the linkage between socioeconomic status and survival. Concentrating on a population where the major differences are socioeconomic rather than racial, the SLACS provides some of the required information.

Income, Education, and Survival: The SLACS Findings

Scientists are reasonably sure that *something* related to the cancer patient's social class affects his or her survival chances. But what is it about the person's position that really makes the difference? In view of the observation that, at least in the United States, a person's class boils down to a set of distinct individual characteristics—income, education, prestige, etc.—the exploration of specific aspects of class is especially important. Income, education, prestige, wealth, culture, and other individual items falling under the rubric of class may, moreover, affect cancer survival in different ways.

The SLACS has important capabilities for helping improve understanding in this area. Previous studies had access mainly to information found in medical records. Thus, they inferred the patient's class position from his or her race or residence. Such an inference is often inaccurate, because an individual patient may be substantially better or worse off than his or her neighbors. The SLACS, however, obtained specific information on income, education, and other dimensions of stratification from individuals. The study, moreover, involved not a particular hospital or clinic but a diverse sample of patients from an entire geographical area.

To view the "big picture," the SLACS researchers began by dissecting the concept of social class. As most American social scientists do today, they addressed social class as a set of specific characteristics that do not necessarily coalesce in the same individual. These *dimensions of social stratification,* a more appropriate term than *class* in this type of study, included income, education, prestige, and wealth.

The researchers obtained information on each patient's level of education and family income in face-to-face interviews. They determined prestige by looking at the patient's occupation—either the one at which he or she now worked or, for the retired, the usual occupation he or she pursued during the working years. Wealth—money in the bank, stocks and bonds, real estate, and the like—was assessed on the basis of the patient's neighborhood. People who live in the same neighborhood usually occupy very similar social positions. Because a person's house is often his or her most important asset, value of the houses in a person's neighborhood may constitute a useful (though not infallible) indication of his or her overall wealth.

The researchers ran all this information through a statistical sifting process, to decide whether multiple dimensions are really important for providing an overview, and, if so, which should receive the most attention. Income and education proved to be the most important of the social-stratification dimensions. Once these facts were known about a patient, prestige and wealth added little to researchers' ability to predict longevity. Having made this determination, the researchers developed a socioeconomic-status index, which captured the individual's income and education under one label. Details of the rationale and procedures for constructing this index appear in Appendix B.

Based on this index, Figure 7 provides an overview of the relationship between socioeconomic status and five-year survival among individuals with lung, prostate, and cervical cancer. Figure 7 reflects differences in survival between the lowest- and highest-scoring patients on the socioeconomic-status index. All patients were placed in one of four categories according to their index scores, the 25 percent lowest-scoring falling into the lowest category, the next 25 percent in the next lowest, and so on. Figure 7 compares patients in the lowest category with those in the highest 25 percent. As in earlier phases of the analysis, the SLACS researchers controlled for age, sex, and cancer site. In examining social class, they added place of residence (rural versus urban), a factor potentially affecting access to health care, as a control.

Generally, people in the higher categories seem more likely to survive five years than those in the lowest category. When all cancers are combined, people in the highest three categories—those with the highest combination of dollars of family income and years of schooling—all appear more likely to survive than those in the lowest category. But this

Those with high status have the best odds.

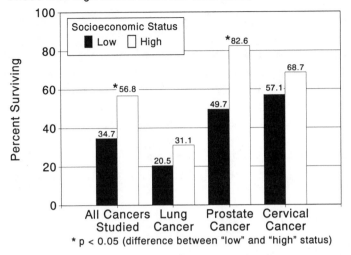

Fig. 7. *Socioeconomic status and five-year survival rates.*

picture is not a consistent one. Figure 7 reflects strong evidence for a survival advantage only for people in the highest income category compared with the lowest. Survival differences between either of the middle categories and the lowest category are not strong enough to rule out the possibility that they may have been observed by chance. This is true for all cancers combined and individual diseases looked at one at a time. Among the individual malignancies, moreover, the difference between the highest and lowest socioeconomic category is strong enough to rule out chance observation only in prostate cancer.

Figure 7 suggests that socioeconomic status, social stratification, or class—whatever label one chooses for position in the social order—has a limited effect on cancer survival. However, since cancer is really a multitude of different diseases and social stratification is a multidimensional phenomenon, the big picture may not be the most meaningful one.

It is important to remember that people in the modern United States may be high on some dimensions of the social-stratification system and low on others. Specific features of an individual's position on the social ladder have different effects on his or her relations with others, behavior, and ability to purchase goods and services. Each of these may, in turn, promote or detract from chances for survival in specific forms of cancer.

INTERMEDIATE STEPS:
DETECTION AND TREATMENT

Both detection and treatment appear to constitute important intermediate steps between class and cancer survival. The individual's position in the social hierarchy should affect detection and treatment, which, in turn, affect survival. Chapter 6 has laid groundwork for further inquiry by indicating the role of early cancer detection, a complex phenomenon in itself, in determining survival.

Tables 3 and 4 examine income and education separately. These tables indicate basic relationships between these dimensions of stratification and specific aspects of early detection and treatment. People on the

Table 3 *Income, Education,*
        and Cancer Detection

In general, high income predicts detection at a routine physical.

	Detected at Routine Physical	
	Income	
	High	*Middle or Low*
All sites	45.3	26.9
Lung	36.8	24.3
Prostate	52.9	28.0
Cervix	33.3	36.3

"All sites" and prostate statistically significant $(p < .01)$

Advanced education also predicts detection at a routine physical.

	Detected at Routine Physical	
	Education	
	College	*Less Than College*
All sites	45.1	27.1
Lung	34.4	25.0
Prostate	53.1	28.3
Cervix	40.4	35.0

"All sites" and prostate statistically significant $(p < .01)$

highest rung of the social ladder are compared with all others. High income is compared with middle and low; college educated is compared with less than college. In this study, it should be noted, high end does not mean elite. High income here means over $35,000, which in Seattle around 1980 was a nice, "middle-class" family income. About 20 percent of those studied here held college degrees.

Tables 3 and 4 suggest that people with higher incomes generally take more prospective action toward early detection than others. For most disease sites, high-income people are more likely to have cancer detected at routine physicals than low- and middle-income people. Those in the

Table 4 *Income, Education, and Cancer Treatment*

High income weakly predicts more intensive treatment.

| | Percentage Receiving Intensive Therapy | |
| | *Income* | |
	High	*Middle or Low*
All sites	40.0	31.0
Lung	44.7	38.7
Prostate	33.3	19.3
Cervix	66.7	31.8

Differences statistically significant only for prostate ($p < .05$)

Advanced education does not predict intensive treatment.

| | Percentage Receiving Intensive Therapy | |
| | *Education* | |
	College	*Less Than College*
All sites	26.4	34.1
Lung	34.4	40.1
Prostate	18.1	24.3
Cervix	40.0	35.0

No differences significant

high-income category are also more likely to receive multimodal treatments—that is, combinations of treatment methods, such as surgery plus radiation, as opposed to surgery alone. Multimodal therapy reflects more intense and aggressive treatment. While many of the relationships involving income in Tables 3 and 4 may have been observed by chance, the relationships between (1) income and detection at a routine physical and (2) income and receiving more intensive treatment are highly consistent.

The relationships between education and intermediate, survival-related phenomena are more specific. A college education appears to be related to having one's cancer detected at a routine physical. As Table 3 shows, this relationship is consistent across the three types of cancers. But education shows no signs of affecting intensity of care.

A more detailed analysis of these relationships, holding key background variables constant, provides more consistent, stronger results. Appendix B gives full details of this analysis and presents resulting statistical tables. The analysis shows the relationships of income and education to intensity of care and detection at a routine physical after age, sex, and residence (rural versus urban), and, in analyses of intensity of care, stage have explained all they can. In addition, this analysis examines a second dimension of early detection (stage at diagnosis) and a second dimension of intensity of care (treatment that includes surgery). In this analysis, the effects of income are presented after those of education have been controlled, and vice versa. Because higher income generally goes along with higher education, it is important to ferret out the independent effects of these dimensions. Finally, the analysis does not merely compare individuals who have high incomes and college degrees with all other individuals; it also assesses the effects of each gradation in earnings and level of schooling on early detection and treatment.

The analysis indicates that the higher a person's family income, the more intensive will be the care he or she receives. For all the malignancies studied here other than lung cancer, the relationships between income and the number of treatment modalities received are positive and strong enough to rule out their having been observed by chance. Both higher incomes and advanced education go along with prospective action related to early detection. When all cancers are looked at together, both income and education coincide with detection of the disease at a routine physical. But on another measure of early detection—the stage at which the disease is finally diagnosed—income and education do not coincide. Instead, a person's level of education provides a better clue than level of income to whether his or her cancer will be detected at early stage.

An examination of the tendency to receive surgery adds complexity to the picture. Surgery is usually an attempt to cure cancer. The surgeon is usually reluctant to operate when a cancer has spread to multiple locations in the body. But surgery also represents an aggressive form of treatment. It is more likely to be a heroic, perhaps last-ditch, attempt at cure than radiation or hormone treatment, which may arrest a disease's progress but does not "cut it out." Surgery is technically intensive and concentrates much expense into a short space of time.

The data indicated no relationship between income and receiving surgery. In a particularly surprising observation, the more education an individual received, the *less* likely he or she was to have been surgically treated. One wonders whether the greater wisdom of the educated makes them avoid this form of treatment. While the picture is complex, this appears to be the basic pattern: (1) more intensive treatment goes along with higher income; (2) earlier detection coincides with both higher income and more years of education.

EFFECTS OF INCOME AND EDUCATION
ON MORTALITY RISK

High intensity of care and early detection are only means to an end. Survival is the bottom line. Does an individual's income or education affect whether he or she will live or die? To answer this question, the SLACS researchers examined the relative mortality risks of people with differing levels of income and education, controlling for several illness-related variables and personal characteristics.

Income. At first glance, income seems to have a weak effect on survival, producing a small survival advantage in each of the forms of cancer examined. In no disease, however, is this relation strong enough to rule out the possibility that it is mere chance observation.

Income has a more definite effect within an important subgroup of lung cancer patients: those who are clinically most likely to benefit from attempted cure. This group encompasses those who have malignancies of the non–small cell type, are diagnosed in Stages I or II, and are sixty-five years old or younger. It is noteworthy that early detection had greater importance for survival among members of this group than for lung cancer patients in general (see Chapter 6). The SLACS researchers found a strong relationship between income and survival within this group. All other things being equal, a higher-income patient of this description had a significantly lower risk of dying over the course of the study than a lower-income patient (an individual with $5,000 less annual family income). It is unlikely that this observation was made by chance.

The researchers were unable to determine why income had this effect. None of the intermediate steps in the detection or treatment process had differed for high- and low-income lung cancer patients. Early detection was not the key. In an analysis that removed the effect of stage, the influence of income became stronger. Whatever gave higher-income people their survival advantage seemed even more important when the influence of stage was removed. All other things being equal, if non–small cell lung cancers of the same stage were detected in two people, the one with the higher income would still have a better survival chance.

Education. When the researchers analyzed data on all the forms of cancer in this study combined, they found that education reduced relative mortality risk. All other things being equal, a given group of patients with one more year of education than another had a 5 percent lower mortality risk. But again, a more detailed look revealed that the effects of education occurred mainly in one form of cancer. The effect of education was strong enough to rule out chance observation only in cancer of the prostate. All things being equal, an additional year of education seemed to increase a prostate cancer patient's chance for survival over the course of the study by almost 12 percent.

Detailed analysis of data on men with prostate cancer suggested at least one reason for this observation. As noted in Chapter 6, an effective method of early detection for prostate cancer was available in the early 1980s: the rectal examination physicians usually perform at routine physicals for men over forty. There is good evidence that early detection results in diagnosis at an earlier stage in prostate cancer. In this study, more years of education were associated with two dimensions of early detection: detection at a routine physical and detection in the absence of pain. The researchers revised their statistical procedure to display the effect of education on survival after these methods of early detection had explained all they could. Education predicted survival less strongly, the strength of the relationship dropping by 25 percent. Part of the connection between education and survival, then, seems to take place through the tendency of people with more education to obtain routine physicals and have their diseases detected in the absence of symptoms. These practices apparently resulted in detection at an early stage, which materially increased survival chances.

But early detection does not tell the whole story. Even after income, detection at a routine physical, detection in the absence of pain, and stage at detection have explained all they can, education continues to reduce mortality risk. Among the more educated men with prostate cancer in this study, something in addition to early detection has taken place which increases survival. The SLACS researchers did not capture this additional phenomenon with their research instruments.

◆　　◆　　◆　　◆　　◆

A detailed analysis reveals that class does indeed affect survival, at least in two of three diseases studied here. The third, cancer of the cervix, is almost certain to behave the same way; it is known to be a true "class" disease, striking poor and black women more often than the affluent and white. The small number of observations of cervical cancer (fifty cases) obtained by the SLACS limited the researchers' ability to perform a definitive analysis.

For the diseases studied here, different mechanisms seem to mediate between specific dimensions of class and survival. Early detection seemed to provide part of the link between education and survival in prostate cancer—a disease for which a reliable, standard early-detection technique existed in the 1980s. Early detection in prostate cancer, however, did not explain the entire effect of education on survival. Early detection played *no* role in the association between income and survival in non–small cell lung cancer. This is not entirely surprising. While early detection appears to have contributed to survival in *some* non–small cell lung cancer cases, physicians had no readily available, sure method for early detection at the time patients in the study were diagnosed. While the SLACS demonstrates a relationship between class and cancer survival, then, the reasons for this relationship remain, in part, a mystery.

How much of the advantage evidenced by relatively well-off people can be explained by diffuse factors such as the patients' assertiveness, support at home, compliance with medical regimens, general self-care, management of complications, nutrition, better interpersonal relations with health professionals, access to more skilled physicians, or better hospitals? This study can make only a few educated guesses. Some people in high-class positions survive longer because they obtain routine physicals. Better access to high-quality and perhaps more intense medical care may also contribute to their relative advantage, as may better advice about the benefits and hazards involved in specific treatment choices.

The mechanism by which class affects cancer survival appears to differ from malignancy to malignancy. But the fact that people in lower-class positions generally have poorer prospects for survival should alarm those who prize the image of the United States as a society that provides its members with equal protection from common hazards. Of even greater concern should be the possibility that increasing numbers of Americans may soon encounter problems once restricted to the poor in obtaining early detection and appropriate treatment for cancer.

CHAPTER EIGHT

The Health Maintenance Organization: A Model for the Future?

The health maintenance organization (HMO) may represent the future of medicine in the United States. This method of providing health care constitutes a sharp departure from American traditions. The HMO embodies the transformation of medicine from a small-office profession with a "horse and buggy" patina to a modern, high-intensity industry lodged in sprawling facilities and guided by corporate executives and staff marketing experts. Like a plant introduced from afar onto hospitable soil, the HMO established itself in every corner of the land in the late twentieth century. No one knows what its impact on the health and longevity of Americans will be. The HMO's impact on cancer survival constitutes an advance indication.

While perhaps less personal than traditional medicine, the HMO holds forth the potential of diminishing the most important barrier between patient and doctor: cash. When a patient approaches an HMO for service, whether for a simple office visit or a major operation, most of the bill has already been paid. The HMO re-creates in America the essentials of health care as it is delivered in Europe's prosperous democracies. In most of these countries, people receive their health care as a right of citizenship, prepaying for services through their taxes, with the government acting as a large insurance carrier.

Leaders in the HMO movement have argued that the absence of a fee barrier encourages people to see their physicians more regularly, to have suspicious symptoms checked, and to return to the office for follow-up visits. In the context of the preceding chapters, such an effect on the patient's behavior would seem extremely valuable. Discovery of early malignancies in apparently healthy adults is one of the keys to survival. Elimination of immediate expenses associated with cancer may reduce some of the discrepancies between the richer and poorer, the more and less educated.

But the HMO must still be considered an experimental approach to health care delivery in the United States. Authorities have noted that, although the HMO reduces some barriers to patients, it may raise others. Many questions remain unanswered about possible differences in service between the HMO and traditional medicine. As an organization, the HMO continues to evolve, seeking ways to ensure prosperity in an increasingly difficult environment. A careful examination of the history, structure, and performance of the HMO may help determine whether this innovation represents a favorable option for cancer patients now and in the future.

The Rise of the HMO

Sick or well, young or old, nearly every adult American has probably heard of an HMO. Except for health insurance specialists and clinicians, few may recognize the actual label "HMO" or know it as an abbreviation for "health maintenance organization." But the HMO's rise represented one of the most visible changes in the U.S. health care scene in the late twentieth century. Before the 1980s, health care was an important segment of American industry, but it was not particularly visible on a day-to-day basis to those making their living elsewhere and not requiring care. By the late twentieth century, billboards, television, radio, newspapers, and magazines advertised health plans with names like Kaiser, HIP, Maxicare, HealthNet. Almost always, these plans were HMOs.

In essence, the HMO is a health insurance plan that pays benefits in the form of services rather than cash. The subscriber to such a plan—or, more typically, his or her employer—pays premiums. Under traditional plans, an individual who visits a physician or undergoes an operation has his or her bill paid after the fact by an insurer or receives reimbursement for direct payments. Because the health care provider receives payment for each unit of care delivered, the traditional form of health care delivery is often called "fee-for-service." Under the HMO, however, no (or very little) money changes hands except when premiums are paid. The member (or his or her employer) pays a fixed premium, and the HMO provides all care required. Some members—most often, the young and healthy—will utilize few if any services. Others—most notably, those with chronic diseases—will consume large volumes of physician hours, hospital resources, and medications.

Compared with the family doctor of yesteryear, the best-established HMOs look like large business establishments. Unlike the family doctor's home or small office in the community, an HMO may occupy an entire office building with its physicians, paraprofessionals, laboratories, and medical records. A large HMO may operate a chain of such facilities in addition to its own hospitals, and may provide care in several cities and states.

Similarly, today's HMO physician resembles the modern office worker much more closely than did his or her antecedent in community practice. The old-time solo practitioner operated a small business. Support staffing was limited, often restricted to the physician's wife (medicine in the United States was almost exclusively a male profession before the 1970s). The traditional physician worked long hours—at least partly because, under the fee-for-service payment system, his income increased with each test or treatment he performed. The doctor was his own boss, typically having the last word in the care of his patients. In the absence of serious misconduct, no outsider intervened. If the family doctor could not perform a needed operation or other type of service, he referred the patient to a colleague with whom he maintained personal ties. Such ties served as channels to keep the family doctor informed of the specialist's level of competence. They also ensured that the patient would see a specialist who would refrain from commenting on errors he might detect in the community physician's work and who would send the patient back to him when specialized treatment was concluded.

More like a modern office worker than an old-time small businessman, the HMO physician does not necessarily increase his or her income by working more intensely or putting in more hours. At an HMO, all patients (or their sponsors) pay a fixed fee in advance. Traditionally, the HMO physician receives a salary. In the absence of advantages to be gained from seeing more patients or performing more procedures, the HMO physician works shorter hours than the fee-for-service practitioner.[1] While primary care physicians in HMOs—family practitioners, general internists, and pediatricians, who provide most day-to-day care—earn about the same income as their fee-for-service counterparts, specialists such as gynecologists, urologists, and surgeons may earn less in the HMO than they would on the outside.[2]

The absence of the virtual autonomy traditionally enjoyed by physicians is also an important distinction. The modern HMO physician always has someone looking over his or her shoulder. Most HMOs maintain peer-review committees of various types to monitor the quality of each physician's practice.

Perhaps most important, HMOs carefully monitor features of the physician's practice that may raise costs. HMOs typically apply mechanisms designed to discourage physicians from performing procedures that may be unnecessary—mechanisms ranging from informal oversight by administrators to payment of cash bonuses for practicing in an economical manner. Most HMOs restrict the family doctor in referring patients to specialists, allowing referrals only to specialists working for the same HMO. Cost-control mechanisms of this kind are crucial for the HMO's survival. HMOs receive no additional income for performing additional services and no additional compensation if their costs rise unexpectedly. HMOs usually project annual costs for treating patients and set premium levels based on these projections. They risk losing considerable amounts of money if they provide more services than anticipated or if the services cost more than expected. On the other hand, the HMO makes money if it provides less treatment or operates more economically than anticipated at the beginning of the year. Thus, the HMO's success depends on applying incentives to its physicians to discourage avoidable visits, procedures, prescriptions, or referral to specialists.

In view of the HMO's visibility and departures from traditional health care delivery, it is surprising to realize that such organizations have existed for many years and stem from pedestrian ancestors. Many small operations offering unlimited medical care on a prepaid basis existed throughout the nineteenth century. It is not uncommon to meet a hospital administrator who proudly boasts that his or her hospital developed the "first HMO," back in the 1800s. The idea of comprehensive medical services in exchange for prepaid fees seems to have been particularly appropriate for industries such as railroad construction and logging, which were isolated from cities and towns. Both managers and unions found physicians willing to follow the camps and provide service in exchange for the steady income made available by prepayment.

Large, modern HMOs began to emerge in the middle of the twentieth century. Kaiser Permanente became perhaps the best known of these plans, enrolling millions of subscribers throughout the United

States. The plan draws its name from industrialist Henry J. Kaiser. A giant in American industrial history, Kaiser served as a major contractor for government projects such as the Depression-era Grand Coulee Dam and World War II shipbuilding on the West Coast. The large labor forces under Kaiser's supervision had difficulty obtaining medical care in the isolated regions where dam construction took place or in the doctor-scarce World War II years. Kaiser arranged for low-cost insurance for his workers and retained a medical group, headed by physician Sidney Garfield, to provide medical care on a prepaid basis.[3] While much larger in scope, the Kaiser plan shared essential characteristics with prepaid arrangements made for isolated, mobile work forces in earlier times.

The Kaiser plan opened its doors to the general public after the war ended. Two administrative and contracting units with the same board of directors, the Kaiser Foundation Health Plan and the Kaiser Foundation Hospitals, enroll patients, maintain records, operate facilities, and contract with physicians to provide services.[4] Medical services are usually provided by the Permanente medical groups, independent partnerships or professional corporations that contract exclusively with the plan. The Kaiser plan blossomed in the post–World War II era, enrolling millions in burgeoning California and initiating new plans in other rapid-growth areas throughout the United States. Organizationally stable, free from debt, able to restrain premium increases, and enjoying a favorable public image, the Kaiser plan became the best-established HMO in the United States.

Other large HMOs of similar vintage have not always achieved comparable success. Like the Kaiser plan, the Health Insurance Plan (HIP) of Greater New York emerged as a response to Depression-era concerns over availability of medical care. While Henry J. Kaiser sought to remove geographical barriers to health care facing his workers, New York mayor Fiorello H. La Guardia, a prime mover in the development of the HIP, was concerned with economic barriers. On the basis of experiments with prepaid plans for the poor, the city government and unions collaborated in developing the prepaid health plan, which began operation in 1947.[5]

In contrast to Kaiser Permanente, HIP owned none of its facilities; it contracted with numerous medical groups, whose members usually devoted most of their attention and effort to private practice. This decentralized structure weakened individual commitment to the plan and the plan's ability to monitor operations and respond to dissatisfaction expressed by plan members. Brown describes several consequences that had become apparent by the mid-1950s: "For many [HIP] physicians, administrators and members remarked despondently, HIP was a hobby, a sop to charity medicine, a means of assuring a stable income while launching a private practice, an attractive side income, or something untaxing to do while easing into retirement. Rumors of second-class care made their way along various grapevines. A familiar anecdote told of physicians who insisted that HIP patients sit in their private waiting rooms until all fee-for-service patients had been seen."[6]

The large HMOs of the post–World War II era had to overcome bitter opposition from the medical establishment. During much of the twentieth century, the American Medical Association (AMA) opposed any and all developments that it considered a deviation from the accepted tradition. These deviations included a broad range of innovations that are accepted everywhere today, such as corporate practice of medicine, health insurance—and HMOs.[7] Evoking the Cold War rhetoric of the 1940s and 1950s, the AMA branded HMOs a form of "socialized medicine," implying that their establishment was a step toward life under a Communist dictatorship, or at least the bleak standard of living tolerated by an impoverished Europe.

The establishment of large-scale HMOs in the United States required a series of victories in court. County medical societies, the local units of the AMA, made professional life very difficult for physicians who joined or collaborated with HMOs. Such physicians were expelled from or denied membership in the county medical societies and, as a result, were isolated professionally and lost admitting privileges to local hospitals.[8] A landmark Supreme Court decision, *American Medical Association v. United States,* found the AMA and an important county medical society guilty of antitrust violations for these practices and levied fines on both. Similar legal struggles and informal disputes between HMOs and the AMA continued for years, however.

The HMO might have retained a small, specialized niche in American health care had it not been for an important government initiative in the early 1970s. Senator Edward Kennedy, for a time the Democrat most favored to challenge President Richard Nixon in 1972, advocated a tax-supported national health insurance program. To deprive Kennedy of a potentially powerful issue in the 1972 race, the Nixon administration chose to support the expansion of HMOs as a solution to the "health care crisis." This initiative resulted in the Health Maintenance Organization Act of 1973 (PL 93-222). The law included a provision requiring employers with twenty-five or more employees who offered health insurance as a benefit to include an HMO as an option if one was available and asked to be offered. This requirement led to a massive increase in the formation of HMOs throughout the United States.

Government policy encouraged vigorous competition among the new HMOs. The Reagan administration enthusiastically embraced competition as a means of controlling health care costs. Under the Reagan administration, HMOs were encouraged to bid for contracts to serve the beneficiaries of massive government-supported health care programs such as Medicare and Medicaid. New state laws allowed private health insurance companies (including HMOs) to bid competitively for hospital services. Because they were large in comparison with most medical practices and had professional, central management structures, the HMOs were at a distinct advantage in establishing a competitive strategy.

While advertising to the public is the most visible manifestation of competition among HMOs, the most important activity in this area may take place behind closed doors. HMOs usually do not seek to enroll members on an individual basis. Instead, they approach employers to offer their plans to their employees. HMOs prefer members who are gainfully employed, because these individuals are usually in better health than the population in general. Younger, healthier people place the HMOs at lower risk of having to provide a higher volume of service than they anticipate. Employers like HMOs because they provide a wide range of services under a single contract. In addition, by offering this range of services under a fixed price agreed upon in advance, the HMO allows an employer to calculate its costs for employee health care in advance, reducing a major business uncertainty. In a given year, any large employer will receive bids from several HMOs competing for the right to enroll its employees.

It is ironic that as America became more conservative in the late twentieth century, it turned to the HMO to help solve its problems in ensuring an affordable health care system. Physicians and other critics may have called HMOs socialized medicine in the 1950s; but by the 1980s, health professionals of all political persuasions referred to HMOs as a form of "managed care"—a term designating a system in which a third party, standing between patient and physician, has the power to question the necessity of care and monitor, reduce, or even entirely disallow charges for services. Cold War rhetoric, which branded HMOs as socialistic in the 1950s, was replaced by business jargon, which characterized the organizations as appropriately "managed" services in the 1980s.

The rapid rise of the HMO and its nontraditional style of functioning raise many questions. For all its faults, the traditional physician-patient relation underscores the physician's personal responsibility to the patient, and materially rewards him or her for performing well. The HMO, on the other hand, faces intense pressure to contain costs; therefore, according to some critics, it may be unable to maintain quality. Like the HIP patients described above, HMO members have always complained about time in the waiting room and the absence of that personal touch attributed to the old-time family doctor. Observers must ask whether HMOs restrict only unnecessary care or cross the crucial boundary between services that may be omitted and those that the patient genuinely needs. This question is especially critical for cancer. The patient has the best chance of survival if diagnosis is timely and accurate, and treatment appropriate. If a health care provider restricts the resources necessary to accomplish these goals, needless mortality may result.

Quality of Care in the HMO

Those concerned with the quality of health care in the United States today and in the future must critically examine the positives and negatives of the HMO. Observers sometimes question the label "health maintenance organization." Research has not established that HMOs maintain health, in the sense that they prevent illness or meet their members' continuing needs better than more traditional health care providers. Evidence has in fact surfaced that while HMOs do a better job for some individuals, they may do a poorer job for others. It is, moreover, important to examine the HMO not as it was in the past or is today, but as it is likely to function in the future, given the competitive pressures it will continue to face.

A sidelight of HMO growth in the era discussed above was the popularization of the term *HMO* itself. Specialists in health care delivery had traditionally referred to this type of system as "prepaid group practice." The term *HMO* was invented by Dr. Paul Elwood, an important health care official in the Nixon administration. The new term differed from the older, neutral designation of a specific type of delivery system by implying favorable outcomes. Elwood and other HMO supporters suggested that by eliminating the fee barrier, prepaid group practice encouraged treatment of disease at an early stage, when its management was presumably easier and less costly in both material resources and human suffering.

While logical, this reasoning is open to criticism. HMOs have earned the attention they have received by eliminating the fee barrier to care. But HMOs must and do erect other barriers to access. Queuing is an important barrier to care in the HMO. A term used by efficiency experts to denote waiting for the availability of a resource, queuing occurs to some degree in most health care systems. In view of the emphasis that has been placed on the early detection of cancer, queuing as a means of restricting access to care has special importance.

Some mechanism of access restriction is crucial in an HMO. An organization providing a service without immediate, direct cost to the consumer would be faced with a burdensome volume of requests for care if it did not erect such barriers. Thus, HMOs may require patients to wait for care longer than fee-for-service providers—either for the scheduling of appointments or in the waiting room itself. Since many illnesses go away on their own in the absence of medical intervention, a waiting period does reduce the eventual volume of service requests. However, the question remains whether some patients will delay seeking care for which they have a vital need.

HMO managers use other methods to restrain the volume and cost of services. Cost advantages may be gained if specialized facilities and personnel are kept in relatively short supply. An oversupply of hospital beds and surgical specialists, for example, is a major concern in the health care industry today. Some administrators have reported that HMOs maintain fewer hospital beds and employ fewer specialists per enrolled population than fee-for-service providers in the surrounding community. Such a policy would reduce costs, because these beds and specialists go through periods of low utilization, during which overhead and salaries must still be paid. But in times of high utilization, the HMO may have to delay care for even those in need.

Physicians themselves may respond to the HMO environment in ways that adversely affect patients with undetected disease. As noted above, the HMO physician does not usually increase his or her income by seeing more patients, and thus has no monetary incentive to increase working hours. The physician is more likely to manage a crowded schedule by spending less time with each individual patient. Such behavior may reduce the patient's ability to relax and discuss his or her concerns with the physician. Technical consequences are possible as well. In his study of a prepaid group practice, Freidson reports the comments of one physician, "'I'm continually irritated at the lack of time, that I don't have enough time to do the kind of work that I want to do. I like to talk to people and I don't have time to do that unless I cut corners. . . . I cut corners by cutting out talking and cutting out the social history, and the social history, for an internist, at least, gives a key to at least half his diagnosis.'"[9] Freidson himself comments that this behavior may have "some bearing on the technical quality of care, for occasional skipping of elements of medical routine may have led to missing conditions at an early stage, when their treatment might have been easier and surer."[10]

These comments suggest that HMOs do not just economize by making patients wait longer for care, but actually deliver a different style of care—one that restricts the volume of resources, such as physician time, allocated to each patient. An important review of the practices of HMOs through the early 1970s adds evidence to this belief. Reviewing several important studies, Luft concluded that there was "clear evidence that total medical-care costs are lower for HMO enrollees than for comparable people with conventional health insurance."[11] In an observation of major impact, Luft traced these cost "savings" to a consistent characteristic of the HMOs he studied: these providers clearly tended to hospitalize their patients less frequently, and when patients did enter the hospital, they stayed fewer days. Hospital stays account for a major portion of health care expenditures today.

Luft's observation does not indicate that HMO patients necessarily receive inferior services. Today many procedures that were once restricted to the hospital setting, ranging from involved diagnostic tests to surgery, are performed in doctors' offices or other outpatient facilities. But critical observers note that the HMO's reluctance to hospitalize may have serious drawbacks. The lower hospitalization rate may reflect restriction of potentially beneficial procedures. It is often said that patients today are being discharged from hospitals "quicker and sicker" than in the past—indicating that shorter stays may deny the patient sufficient time to recover from procedures performed in the hospital or to regain function after episodes of acute illness.

Early studies of HMOs supported the belief that they produce more favorable health outcomes for their members than the fee-for-service providers available to them. In the 1950s and 1960s, a group of researchers performed several studies to compare health outcomes of those receiving care from HIP and from fee-for-service providers in Greater New York. These studies reported lower rates of premature birth, infant mortality, and mortality among the poor and elderly in the HIP.[12] But, because the studies did not take certain factors into account, the favorable outcomes observed cannot be clearly attributed to the HMO. People who joined HIP, for example, often enjoyed advantages, in the form of stable employment and income, over those who did not join.[13] Those who joined may have been more concerned with safeguarding their personal health. Both these factors are capable of explaining the more favorable health outcomes observable among HIP members.

The 1970s brought more definitive studies utilizing highly sophisticated research designs. The Rand Health Insurance Study was most important in this area. Unlike perhaps any other research effort before or since, the Rand study had an experimental design. The study selected people from several major metropolitan areas and randomly assigned them to different types of insurance plans. Some of the experimental subjects in Seattle, Washington, one of the metropolitan areas in the Rand study, were assigned to Group Health Cooperative of Puget Sound—an HMO important in the SLACS as well.[14] The Rand study had advantages over all preceding research on HMOs, because it compared individuals in an HMO and a fee-for-service setting who were similar in all other respects.

The Rand study generally confirmed findings of earlier researchers with respect to utilization of services in an HMO versus fee-for-service. HMO patients were less likely to be hospitalized than those in fee-for-service, but more likely to make visits to their physicians' offices over a given period of time.[15] The Rand study also compared outcomes of care for HMO and fee-for-service patients according to a wide variety of measures. Among poor people who began the study with established health problems, those in the HMO had worse health outcomes according to two measures than those who received free care in a fee-for-service setting. Specifically, poor people were more likely to experience disability and had greater risks of mortality than their counterparts in "free" fee-for-service.[16]

Few studies have been made of cancer patients in HMOs. In one such study, an investigation of terminal cancer patients in New York State in the late 1970s and early 1980s, patients in three HMOs were compared with those in fee-for-service. The investigators found no differences in the dimensions they examined: hospital admissions, days of hospitalization, and costs.[17] Another study, focusing on colorectal cancer patients, compared the services and outcomes of care obtained by members of Group Health Cooperative of Puget Sound (the same HMO as observed in the RAND study) with fee-for-service patients in the surrounding community. The study compared 39 HMO patients with 150 fee-for-service and monitored their survival for up to four years.[18] The HMO patients made more physicians' office visits and received more endoscopy examinations than their fee-for-service counterparts. Both groups were equally likely to receive surgery, radiation, or chemotherapy. Of particular interest was the finding that the HMO patients waited longer between first contact with their physicians and the beginning of treatment. But the researchers found no difference between the survival times observed for the two groups.

A highly visible and radical departure from traditional health care, HMOs have attracted considerable attention from researchers. Generally, the HMO studies suggest that these organizations provide a style of care different from that of traditional medicine. Services tend to emphasize ambulatory care, with fewer and shorter hospitalizations but more frequent office visits—although these appear more likely to be rushed than office visits in a fee-for-service setting. Conclusions with respect to outcomes have been mixed. Questions about the possible effects of the HMO structure on the quality of services and the appropriate role for HMOs in the United States health care system remained unresolved in the late twentieth century.

Group Health Cooperative: A Landmark HMO

Time and place provided the SLACS researchers with an unusual opportunity to study the impact of HMO treatment on cancer survival. Performing their research in the Seattle metropolitan area, they were able to include among their subjects many patients belonging to Group Health Cooperative of Puget Sound, the same HMO studied in the famous RAND project. The SLACS researchers, then, could follow patients from the time their cancers were diagnosed until the patients died or the study ended, and compare those in the HMO with those in fee-for-service. Unlike the RAND investigators, researchers in the SLACS were unable to use an experimental design. However, they were able to use statistical techniques to take account of factors that might cover up or explain away the relationship between HMO membership and cancer survival. The researchers were especially fortunate to have begun their study in the early 1980s. At that time, Group Health

Cooperative was the only HMO operating in the Seattle-Tacoma area. Thus, any person not identified as a member could be presumed to receive his or her care from a fee-for-service provider.

The structure, history, and values of Group Health Cooperative make it a true landmark in the HMO movement. In many ways, it represents the ideal HMO—even more than Kaiser Permanente, which has much larger enrollments, or the HIP, which is older. All Group Health Cooperative physicians, first, are salaried employees who work only for the cooperative. This arrangement differs not only from the traditional independent practitioner, group practice, and professional corporation that dominate fee-for-service, but from Kaiser Permanente as well. At least in California, where Kaiser's largest operations take place, physicians join a professional corporation that provides services only to Kaiser. Although these physicians are not the independent small businesspeople of old, they are not employees either. In employing physicians directly, Group Health Cooperative breaks completely with tradition.

Group Health Cooperative's history represents a paradigm of HMO origins and development. The organization's roots are visible in the self-help and cooperative movements that became popular in the Pacific Northwest in the early twentieth century. Its history also reflects the desire among people all over the United States to reform social institutions in the post-Depression era. Group Health shares and in some respects typifies the history of intense conflict between the HMO and establishment medicine.

Group Health Cooperative has clear links with the organizations established by Northwest farmers and loggers to provide mutual assistance and obtain medical services in isolated locations. As World War II drew to a close, leaders in Washington State's consumer cooperatives, unions, and Granges began searching for a means of providing reliable, prepaid health care to their members and the community. Resources capable of providing this care came in the form of an eighteen-physician group practice called the Medical Security Clinic, which the fledgling Group Health Cooperative purchased in 1946 for $200,000. The clinic itself had specialized in providing prepaid care: its precursor organization (the Western Clinic and Hospital Association in Tacoma) served loggers through prepayments deducted from their salaries since 1916, and prospered on contracts with Seattle-area defense industries during World War II.[19]

Conflict with established medicine almost immediately followed the cooperative's formation. As was typical in this era, the King County

Medical Society (the American Medical Association's local unit) barred Group Health Cooperative physicians from membership, characterizing prepaid practice as unethical per se. Rejection by the county medical society meant cancellation of admitting privileges to hospitals other than the small facility owned by Group Health itself, exclusion from continuing medical education, and general professional ostracism. In 1949, Group Health Cooperative sued the King County Medical Society, charging the organization with conspiracy in restraint of trade. The cooperative initially lost its case in Superior Court but won on appeal in 1951.

Following these milestone events, Group Health Cooperative struggled through internal conflicts and financial crises into the 1950s. Membership grew slowly, numbering a few thousand by the middle of the decade. But as the Puget Sound area boomed in the 1960s and 1970s, and the HMO Act of 1973 encouraged employers to offer membership to employees, enrollment exploded, reaching 330,000 by the 1980s, about 15 percent of the area's population—respectable market penetration in today's management jargon.

Group Health Cooperative's extensive physical facilities, large membership, and accepted status in the 1980s contrast with its humble origins. The organization boasts an array of large hospital and clinic buildings in metropolitan Seattle, and satellite facilities in the sprawling suburban areas and across the Cascade Mountains in eastern Washington. Often in collaboration with the University of Washington, Group Health Cooperative conducts world-class research.

But, as in any system so different from traditional medicine, quality of care remains an issue. Old-line members express pride in the cooperative's success and praise its service. But others grumble about "assembly line medicine"; some tell stories about receiving desired treatment only after extraordinary efforts. Not surprisingly, some fee-for-service physicians in the surrounding community question Group Health Cooperative's ability to provide patients with the best care technology has to offer.

Cancer Treatment and Survival in the HMO and Fee-for-Service

Do these and related complaints merely reflect a long-established tendency of Americans to deprecate those who provide them with health care, whatever the setting, or to hark back to an imagined past where a kindly family doctor provided personalized, low-cost attention? Or does the discomfort reflect problems that go beyond cosmetics and trappings that a large HMO may fail to provide? Part of the answer is provided by a comparison of services and survival chances of Group Health Cooperative members with those of their neighbors in fee-for-service.

The SLACS researchers made these comparisons on the basis of the three cancers most amenable to medical intervention in their investigation: lung, prostate, and cervix. Patient characteristics other than HMO membership that were known to affect, or were suspected of affecting, health care utilization or outcomes (income, education, living outside an urban area, etc.) were controlled. As in earlier chapters, details about the analysis and specific statistical findings are presented in Appendix B.

The investigators first compared the process of care and the types of services patients received in the HMO and fee-for-service settings. Stage at diagnosis, the crucial factor in forecasting how long a patient could be expected to live, did not differ much in the two settings; chance alone could have explained the observed difference. Nor was there a statistically significant difference between HMO and fee-for-service patients in the amount of time that passed between their discovery of a symptom and the delivery of a diagnosis. HMO members did experience more delay in treatment. On the average, they waited about two weeks longer than fee-for-service patients from the time their physicians made diagnoses of cancer until they began receiving treatment. This difference was too large to suggest that it was caused only by chance. While the HMO may have acted less rapidly than the fee-for-service system in starting treatment, however, it did not appear to treat patients less intensively. The researchers made two comparisons of intense forms of care as received by HMO and fee-for-service patients: surgical and multimodal treatment. They detected no differences large enough to rule out the possibility that they were observed by chance.

Most important, of course, is whether the HMO member's chance of survival is greater or less than that of the person receiving fee-for-service care. As reported in earlier chapters, the researchers assessed chances of survival by examining both five-year survival and relative risk of dying (HMO versus fee-for-service patients) over the course of the study. When all individuals in the study were examined at the same time, those in the HMO seemed to have a somewhat better chance of surviving five or more years after diagnosis than those in fee-for-service; but the magnitude of the difference left open the possibility that it was observed by mere chance. The relative risk over the course of the study was lower for HMO members than for fee-for-service patients, but the difference was still inconclusive. Moreover, when specific types of cancer were examined individually, the apparent effects of HMO membership were not consistent. HMO patients with lung and cervical cancers seemed to have poorer survival chances than their fee-for-service counterparts. The availability of only three HMO members with cervical cancer in the SLACS sample limited the study's analytical power for this site, although HMO membership predicted a lower survival probability over the course of the study. HMO members with prostatic cancer, however, had a *better* chance of surviving five years and a lower relative risk than those in fee-for-service—a statistically significant result. These findings, summarized in the top panel of Figure 8, suggest no overall effect of HMO membership.

When the researchers asked whether HMO membership had different effects among people with high and low incomes, they obtained results that were considerably more distinct. The researchers divided the SLACS patients into three categories based on family income: low (less than $20,000 per year); middle (between $20,000 and $34,999); and high ($35,000 or over). Individuals in the HMO who reported low family incomes seemed to obtain a distinct advantage over patients with similar incomes in fee-for-service. Figure 8 (bottom panel) indicates that low-income patients treated in the HMO had a greater chance of surviving for five years after diagnosis than low-income fee-for-service patients. Low-income HMO members had about half as great a chance of dying over the course of the study as those in fee-for-service. The differences between low-income patients in fee-for-service and the HMO are large enough to suggest strongly that they were not observed by chance. In all the cancers covered in this study, moreover, low-income HMO patients experienced higher five-year survival and a lower relative death risk over the course of the study than low-income fee-for-service patients.

Although the "average" patient, then, appears to have about the same chance of survival and life expectancy whether treated in the HMO or fee-for-service, the low-income patient seems to gain an advantage by obtaining care in the HMO. The researchers tried to discover reasons for this advantage. More rapid detection or more intensive care could not explain the difference, because the HMO members seemed to receive similar care, and certainly moved no sooner into treatment. The investigators asked whether the HMO achieved its apparent advantages for people of limited means principally because it allowed them to receive

Generally, HMO members do not seem to do better or worse.

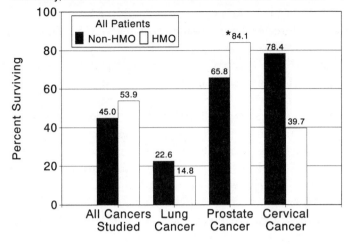

But low-income patients obtain some advantages.

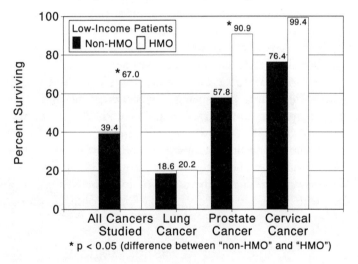

* p < 0.05 (difference between "non-HMO" and "HMO")

Fig. 8. *HMO membership and five-year survival rates.*

care without paying for it out of pocket. When out-of-pocket payment was controlled, however, the advantages for low-income people remained. Moreover, when separate analyses were carried out for people who reported paying at least part of their health care expenses out of pocket and people who reported paying no part, the same results were obtained. This finding is important because some might argue that people in HMOs enjoyed better survival experiences only in comparison with people receiving care from charity providers or public facilities—both of which primarily serve persons in extreme poverty and are likely to demand no payment. Highly similar results were obtained in comparisons of (1) HMO members and persons in fee-for-service who paid at least part of their health care bills and (2) HMO members and fee-for-service patients who paid nothing. Thus, it appears that people in the low-income category who belonged to the HMO had better chances of survival not because they were less likely to be "charity cases" than low-income people in fee-for-service but because of something positive that the HMO contributed to their care.

The SLACS was unable to explain the HMO's benefit for low-income people or, for that matter, to indisputably attribute increased survival to better *cancer management* in the HMO. Persons with generally better health may have tended to select the HMO, consistent with a belief that they should adopt a lifestyle cognizant of the possibility of serious illness and concerned with its prevention. It is also possible that the observed survival differences are explained by better management of illnesses other than cancer in the HMO than in fee-for-service settings. Even if both of these possibilities were proven true, however, the HMO could still be said to benefit cancer patients in the low-income category. The HMO would prove beneficial, first, by enabling low-income people with the motivation to care for themselves to do so and, second, by providing them with better care for the conditions that accompany chronic disease.

The HMO: A Sign of Progress?

It seems likely that the HMO neither increases nor decreases survival chances for most cancer patients. But, at least in Group Health Cooperative of Puget Sound in the 1980s, there appeared to be some definite winners. These were patients economically disadvantaged relative to others observed in the SLACS—a factor that would have placed them in an inferior position if they had had to shop for health care in the open market, cash in hand.

Were there also losers? Did HMO membership constitute a disadvantage for the more affluent, who are better able to purchase the best health care available on the open market? Because HMOs rarely cover care outside the plan, these patients might be discouraged from searching elsewhere for treatment options more appropriate for their individual conditions. The SLACS found no evidence of a disadvantage for the more affluent. However, an examination of diseases other than lung, prostate, and cervical cancer might yield other results, and outcomes in all malignancies should be monitored by future researchers.

It is noteworthy that the SLACS found no specific reason to account for improved survival among those in the lowest third of the income distribution. HMO patients differed from those in fee-for-service neither in the intensity of care they received nor in the stage at which their cancers were diagnosed. Relationships between HMO membership and survival remained after these variables were held constant.

◆   ◆   ◆   ◆   ◆

These findings may encourage support for the HMO as a model for future health care in the United States. It may be argued that the prepayment feature of the HMO removes barriers of key significance to people with limited resources when they need care for a serious, often chronic illness. The SLACS did not indicate a specific reason why the relatively disadvantaged should have survived longer. But the possibility remains that these individuals may have found in the HMO a ready source of care appropriate for their conditions. Treatments in the HMO may have been planned and adjusted according to the needs of individual patients in a more skillful manner than the disadvantaged might ordinarily have obtained in fee-for-service. Better integration among diverse aspects of care, facilitated by the group-practice feature of the HMO, may have helped bring about this result.

But evaluation of this model for future health care must take place with the knowledge that important differences exist among HMOs. Group Health Cooperative, for example, began as a socially progressive organization in a hostile environment. Launched by community activists, opposed by organized medicine, and spurned by banks, it was a far cry from today's new HMOs, organized by professional managers, contracting with established medical groups, and financed through junk bonds. It is quite possible that the "style" of medicine observed in Group

Health Cooperative stems primarily from the unusual physicians it attracted in its early days and their influence on the organization's professional culture.

In addition, HMOs are still evolving—and are doing so in an increasingly competitive environment. After serving as virtually the only alternative to traditional fee-for-service medicine in the Seattle area for a generation, Group Health Cooperative itself began seeing its market invaded by well-financed "managed-care products" of all kinds in the mid-1980s. By aggressively enrolling young working people, those least likely to contract expensive diseases, these competitors were able to offer their services at initially lower prices than Group Health. To safeguard its survival, Group Health Cooperative has departed from some of its most valued traditions.[20] Many members, for example, now pay an out-of-pocket fee for each visit in addition to premiums. A study of the impacts of this fee shortly after its inception indicated that rates of comprehensive physical examinations among female members declined, but not key cancer-screening tests—Pap smear, breast examination, and hemoccult.[21] Of even greater concern are the adaptations that HMOs without Group Health Cooperative's strong traditions may make as competition intensifies. These may prove to be effective business strategies but result in lower quality care.

CHAPTER NINE

Conclusion: Personal Strategies and Public Issues

Cancer will remain a leading concern of all humankind in the foreseeable future and probably well beyond. Everyone faces some risk of developing the disease, no matter how conscientiously he or she applies existing knowledge about prevention. Science will discover no miraculous cures. Few patients will extend their lives by entering experiments. Fewer yet will improve their prospects for survival through psychological approaches or unorthodox care. As individuals, people may materially increase their survival chances by making the most of standard health care. As a society, America in the twenty-first century can best reduce the threat to life that cancer poses by protecting and enhancing the individual's ability to identify, locate, and make use of appropriate health services.

Basing their conclusions on a review of scientific literature and on original research, the preceding chapters call into question many popular beliefs. Consistent with the environmental and fitness movements, many Americans have embraced the concept of cancer prevention. But existing knowledge about environmental and other exogenous factors, as summarized in Chapter 4, suggests that no more than half of the cancers occurring in the United States at the end of the twentieth century could have been prevented; the actual percentage of avoidable cancers was, in fact, probably much lower. Riding the wave of public belief in counseling and self-help, a spate of authors popularized the notion that emotional well-being could cure cancer. But, as detailed in Chapter 5, the research cited by these authors has usually been confined to the petri dish and rodent cage or, when human subjects are used, has been based largely on anecdotes and testimonials. Research that approximates the rigor of biomedical investigations provides no indication that emotional well-being aids physical survival.

The Seattle Longitudinal Assessment of Cancer Survival (SLACS) provides some support for the widely accepted notion that early detection increases the likelihood of survival. Chapter 6 presents evidence that, at least for some forms of cancer, early detection leads to true life extension. But this chapter provides a perspective different from the exhortation to respond to cancer's "seven warning signals." Medical procedures that can detect cancers *before* they produce symptoms visible to the patients seem to be the most valuable.

The relationships detected by the SLACS between personal resources and survival may have the farthest-reaching implications. Cancer patients whose resources seem to help them maintain the most ready access to health care generally survive the longest. Chapter 7 demonstrates that, in cancers where medicine and surgery can make a major difference in survival, higher levels of income and education may correspond to increased life expectancy. Among people with low family incomes, belonging to the right kind of health plan seems to compensate, at least in part, for the lack of ready cash. Chapter 8 indicates that low-income people who received their care through a well-established HMO had better survival chances than their counterparts who paid out of pocket for each doctor visit or hospital stay, or whose sponsors (private insurance companies or the government) paid for their care under such an arrangement.

What actually permits cancer patients with income, educational, and other advantages to survive longer? Early detection appears to tell only part of the story. No connection could be drawn between aggressive treatment and survival. An explanation consistent with the SLACS findings and many earlier studies suggests that the survival advantage arises largely from ready access to skilled practitioners applying widely accepted diagnostic and treatment techniques in well-managed practice settings. These skills and practice conditions are most conducive to accurately determining disease stage, planning therapy, revising treatment in response to changes in the tumor, discovering new facts (as may occur during a surgical procedure), and following patients after initial interventions. Advanced techniques available to a few practitioners in specialized centers only occasionally play a major role in this process. The hallmark of "appropriate care" is skillful application of standard interventions on a case-by-case basis. Achieving, maintaining, and extending access to standard care should be the goal of individuals concerned with reducing the threat of cancer in their own lives and of professionals and policymakers charged with protecting the health and longevity of others.

Individual Survival Strategies: A Consumer Perspective

People may increase their chances of surviving cancer through a practical approach to obtaining quality health care. An effective personal strategy for survival emphasizes establishing networks and mechanisms to facilitate receipt of appropriate care when it is required. Familiar rules for dealing with illnesses in general are important in cancer. These include basics such as learning about therapeutic options and obtaining second opinions. Actions taken before the advent of illness, however, may make the most important difference in an individual's chances for survival. Even the most capable and intelligent people may not make their best decisions when they are sick, frightened, or under pressure to take quick action—conditions that often prevail when cancer is diagnosed.

INFORMED HEALTH CARE SELECTION

Quality varies in all goods and services. Consumers in the late twentieth century have become very sophisticated in their selection of automobiles and home appliances; but they ask fewer questions about doctors, hospitals, and health plans, whose features may make the difference between life and death. People have the right and the responsibility to ask many more questions than they do. Physicians and hospitals vary in their capabilities and the quality of services they provide. As the examples in Chapter 6 illustrate, cancer presents a challenge even to skilled practitioners; misdiagnoses, at least temporary ones, do not appear to be infrequent.

The Physician. The prestige of the medical profession should not deter the prospective patient from asking fundamental questions about a practitioner's background and capabilities. All states require that medical schools be accredited and physicians be licensed. But the licenses of practicing physicians are, in fact, almost never revoked.[1] The person who finishes last in his or her medical school class is still called "doctor."

The primary care physician plays a particularly important role in cancer. It is to this professional that people look for everyday medical care and interpretation of signs of serious illness. The office of every primary care doctor—general internists, family practitioners, gynecologists, pediatricians—should, in fact, be a cancer-detection center. In the event of serious illness, the primary care doctor generally refers the patient to a specialist. While the specialist may perform the actual surgery or chemotherapy in cancer, the primary care physician acts as purchasing agent and "gatekeeper" for these services.

What are the clues to quality in a primary care physician? There are no cookbook formulas. Different physician qualities will vary in importance among consumers. Some may, for example, desire a physician who readily shares a large amount of information with the patient about the reasons for prescribing a certain drug or performing a particular procedure. Others may want to leave this reasoning entirely to the doctor. Everyone, however, should ask where the physician received his or her degree. American medical schools turned out too few physicians for the burgeoning population in the 1950s and 1960s, and came to rely on foreign-trained doctors to fill out the shortage. Doctors from all over the world immigrated to the United States, and today practice everywhere and in every specialty.[2] There is no reason necessarily to avoid a foreign medical graduate; but the patient should recognize that a large number of countries, particularly those of the Third World, have health care systems considerably more primitive than those of the United States and Europe. Their medical schools may reflect these differences.

The wise patient-consumer might also ask about his or her physician's postgraduate education. Virtually all physicians in the United States today complete residencies requiring several years of practical training following medical school. The quality of residency training is at least as important as medical school itself. A residency in a well-known, well-regarded hospital is a good sign. Closely related to residency training is board certification. Most important medical specialties today have boards of professional leaders that monitor residency programs and examine new physicians seeking to practice in their specialty. Obtaining board certification does not necessarily make a man or woman a better doctor. The ability to answer questions on an examination may not translate into better care. But the board-certified physician will have cleared one additional hurdle.

The most important signs of a physician's quality are his or her place in the local medical community and reputation among peers. Medicine is a very social profession; practitioners may be reluctant to talk in public, but they are constantly evaluating each other's skills. The physician who enjoys the highest standing among other physicians and actively communicates with colleagues is generally the best practitioner. Active ties with other leading physicians constitute open channels of communication for the latest medical information. The physician in the highest ranks of his or her medical community will not hesitate to refer a case to another doctor when needed and will select the most skilled consultants.

While doctors rarely evaluate each other publicly, good clues are available to the sophisticated consumer. The prospective patient who has friends or family in the medical community should make use of these ties to gather information. An experienced nurse can provide excellent information about a doctor's reputation among other medical professionals and likely has directly observed how well the patients of individual physicians have done over the years.

The hospitals with which a physician is associated are good clues to his or her professional standing. Before allowing physicians to admit patients to their institution, physicians already practicing at a hospital review the applicant's credentials and reputation. The best medical groups will be the most selective. It seems wise for the consumer to look for a physician who, at minimum, has admitting privileges at one of the leading hospitals in the locality. Most physicians have privileges at several.

Particular criteria should be applied to specialists. The patient referred to a specialist should ask about credentials. A medical license in the United States entitles a physician to practice any specialty; no law restricts a physician from self-designation. For the consumer, however, board certification should be a criterion. Many specialists complete additional graduate work, taking fellowships in subspecialties after they complete their residencies. Thoracic surgery and pediatric oncology are examples. The prospective patient should ask how often the specialist treats a specific cancer, and how often the specialist carries out the actual procedure under consideration. In many forms of medical care, high volume in a specific procedure is an excellent indication of skill and likelihood of success.

Patients in HMOs and other managed-care arrangements should

exercise to the fullest whatever options they have for selecting physicians. The same clues and guidelines proposed above may be applied in an HMO. An HMO may utilize the services of a large number of physicians, and the backgrounds, credentials, and reputations of individuals may vary. Having made his or her selection, of course, the patient may find that the chosen physician is accepting no new patients. In this instance, the patient should have his or her name placed on a waiting list. An HMO physician's practice may include well over a thousand patients. Even among the busiest and most popular, vacancies occur regularly.

The Hospital. The quality of a hospital is a good indication of the standing of the physicians who practice there. The functioning of the hospital itself—the reliability of its laboratories, efficiency of its record keeping, etc.—may make life-or-death differences. To the unsophisticated, all hospitals may look alike. Like HMOs, hospitals today engage in advertising. But, as with most products, commercials provide few objective facts. Those who take the initiative, however, can obtain objective information about a hospital. The Joint Commission on Accreditation of Hospitals, a body including representation from a variety of professional groups, reviews the resources and management of hospitals nationwide. Hospitals must maintain accreditation to receive payments from Medicare and most private insurance plans. Among other criteria, the commission looks for evidence that the hospital exercises regular and conscientious review of the quality of care performed in all its departments. Relatively few hospitals that treat cancer patients lack accreditation. But the strength of an institution will be reflected in the length of its accreditation. The strongest hospitals receive accreditation for three-year terms, the weakest for one year. One-year accreditation may signal probationary status.

Another useful criterion for assessing the quality of a hospital is the percentage of its beds filled on a given day. Most American hospitals in the late twentieth century operated at less than their full capacity. The informed consumer, however, should suspect problems in a hospital that appears to be utilized at a rate below the national average. A hospital with appropriate equipment and support services will retain the loyalty of physicians and attract some of the best; these, in turn, will keep the beds filled. An institution with 40 percent of its beds empty on any given day, however, is probably not of first rank. On a typical day in the late twentieth century, many hospitals in the United States had more than 40 percent of their beds unused.

Patients should realize that many physicians are "splitters," admitting cases to more than one hospital. Physicians may decide where to admit on grounds other than medical ones. The physician may, for example, admit a patient with poorer insurance coverage to a hospital with lower community standing. Like people in other walks of life, the physician may elect to allocate the most desirable resources to his or her most favored partners—doctors and administrators at the hospital of choice. But the patient must always act as his or her own advocate. Among the hospitals where their physician maintains privileges, patients should indicate their own preference, ask why the physician's preference differs (if it does differ), and, after due negotiation, be insistent about their choice.

Like any consumer, patients have rights and should exercise them in a knowledgeable way. The United States no longer has a doctor or hospital shortage; many experts, in fact, believe that a surplus prevails. People should not allow themselves to feel intimidated by the health care system. The questions suggested here need not be asked of the physician directly. A nurse or aide will have information about the physician's credentials and the hospitals to which he or she admits. A few telephone calls to the administrative offices of the hospital should generate information about accreditation and occupancy rates. But the comfort level exhibited by a physician when asked about these matters may be a good indication of his or her professional self-confidence, standing in the medical community, and ability to discuss complex, sensitive information—all important in the process of cancer treatment should it ever become necessary.

The Health Plan. Most people pay only a small fraction of their health care bills out of pocket, carrying insurance to cover most expenses. Employed people usually have an opportunity to select from among several insurance plans. Medicare beneficiaries, who participate in a government insurance program, face difficult choices as well. Many Medicare beneficiaries purchase supplementary insurance to cover services omitted in basic coverage. Typically, these plans differ in cost and services covered. For specific services, an insurance plan may require no copayments; for others, the patient may be required to pay part or all of the cost. HMOs themselves are insurance plans, paying benefits in the form of services instead of cash. They, too, may cover all the cost of some services, and only part or none for others.

Certain features of an insurance plan are particularly important regarding the threat to life and health represented by cancer. Because of the importance of early detection, coverage for routine physical examinations and screening procedures such as mammography may be highly beneficial. In view of the diagnostic and treatment issues that arise in cancer, an appropriately designed health plan would also offer complete or nearly complete coverage for second opinions.

Those considering an HMO or other managed-care product should ask not only about coverage for costs of screening and diagnostic procedures but also about actual availability. How long are the typical waiting times for a mammogram? How frequently does the HMO provide routine physicals? Prospective HMO members should also determine whether the plan would cover the services of specialists outside the HMO should they be needed, and what form of documentation might be required to secure coverage. Some of the best information about these features of an HMO may be obtained from patients who have personal experience with the plan.

While patients may go through this selection process at any time, they gain distinct advantages by acting before they become ill. All things being equal, a healthy person will make better decisions and experience less anxiety in the process than a person with a suspected or confirmed diagnosis of cancer. The most effective consumer in this crucial area will have already completed the process of evaluating and selecting his or her physician, hospital, and health plan by the time cancer or another serious disease strikes. Healthy people should recognize the importance of this process, and not hesitate to carry it out because they have a regular physician to whom they have become accustomed. It is all too easy to become complacent about one's habitual source of medical care, only to find it wanting in the time of greatest need.

PERSONAL RESPONSIBILITY
AND VIGILANCE

Although this book has made much of factors outside the control of the cancer patient, the individual's actions on his or her own behalf remain crucial. Perhaps the most important step a person can take to increase his or her chances of surviving cancer is to have routine medical examinations. While physicians cannot always detect cancer before it produces symptoms, they can do so in many cases. Of all early-detection processes, diagnosis before the advent of symptoms has the highest yield in terms of survival, at least with respect to the cancers studied in this book. People should also take the "seven warning signals" seriously and obtain medical attention upon noticing any of them. But the habit of obtaining routine physicals, while requiring a higher level of awareness and self-discipline, may ultimately be more effective in promoting survival.

Perhaps the most difficult decision in cancer treatment involves refusal of care. The informed patient should objectively evaluate the curative or palliative potential of treatments offered. If offered treatment through a clinical trial, the patient should determine several basic facts. To what phase of the clinical trial process does the proposed treatment belong? In a Phase I trial, the patient will be among the first human beings subjected to the treatment. If human subjects have already received the experimental intervention, what has been their survival experience? What possibility exists that the experimental treatment may shorten life or make the naturally remaining life span less usable or enjoyable?

Public Decisions and Cancer Survival

By emphasizing human behavior and access to resources, the conclusions in this book have focused on nonbiomedical factors affecting the outcomes of a biological condition. This perspective may seem unfamiliar to many, particularly health professionals accustomed to addressing disease in individual human beings. But the importance of these factors merely reflects the general success of humankind's use of technology to overcome the uncertainty of nature. In many areas, technological progress has replaced a struggle between humankind and nature with conflicts over ownership and use of resources. In many parts of the world, fewer and fewer people worry about storms and crop failures, but more and more experience anxiety because of political instability and the business cycle.

Although startling breakthroughs in cancer treatment are unlikely, slow progress will continue. As medicine increases its capabilities, costs will undoubtedly rise. The average cost in 1984 of treating a cancer patient in the United States totaled over $25,000 for the initial and terminal phases alone.[3] Considerably higher costs for futuristic procedures—bone marrow transplant, for example, often exceeded $100,000 in 1990—may be typical in the years to come. For even more cancer patients, access to appropriate care may become problematical at some point during their illness. Along with biomedical progress will come an intensification of nonbiomedical dilemmas.

Cancer survival is, then, both a personal problem and a public issue. Findings in the preceding chapters suggest that *public decisions* may ultimately affect progress in improving cancer survival more profoundly than private ones. Public decisions are those that reflect the collective reasoning and desires of society. They directly and indirectly affect the options open to individuals and the actions they may take. Laws passed by Congress, presidential orders, and Supreme Court actions represent familiar forms of public decisions. Decisions made by insurance industry regulators and public health officials, while less familiar, also are public decisions. Public decisions need not take place in the context of government. Directors of large corporations and union business managers make decisions that affect thousands of consumers and workers. Some public decisions are limited and technical and may be implemented in a straightforward manner. Others are global and normative, requiring redeployment of personal and public resources, changes in key institutions, and revision of basic values. Public decisions on both levels affect cancer survival.

LIMITED DECISIONS

Public decisions of a limited technical nature can affect the survival chances of many individuals. The most familiar of these decisions have addressed environmental hazards. Most jurisdictions in the United States have adopted laws limiting the use of asbestos and ordering its removal from schools and other public buildings. Laws governing food additives suspected of causing cancer have already been discussed. These laws may have major consequences for governments and industries. By the beginning of the twenty-first century, the bill facing American municipalities for asbestos abatement may reach $100 billion. Still, existing statutes and regulations governing hazardous environmental substances do not challenge basic American values. They rest on a firm foundation of belief in government's role as guardian of the public safety.

Public decision-making in this limited sense may solve some of the problems raised in the preceding chapters. Tighter regulation of cytology laboratories processing Pap smear slides and other tests related to cancer detection, for example, would certainly prevent some avoidable mortality. Public oversight of most health professions, an established fact throughout the twentieth century, and periodic examination of hospitals by the Joint Commission on Hospital Accreditation are precedents for such regulation. Similarly, state insurance commissions could mandate that procedures for early detection of cancer be included in health insurance plans. Such provisions, already part of Washington State's insurance regulatory code in 1990, seem likely to appear in many other jurisdictions in the years to come.

Issues surrounding tobacco suggest a boundary for limited public decision-making of this kind. Without question, tobacco represents the greatest known exogenous cancer hazard. Strong arguments exist for severely restricting its marketing, packaging, and advertising. Public decisions, including voluntary actions by employers and advertisers, have greatly restricted where tobacco can be sold and used. But the value Americans place on personal liberty will probably prevent serious consideration of an outright ban.

GLOBAL ISSUES

The importance of access to appropriate care in cancer survival raises more profound questions for American society in the twenty-first century. As was pointed out in the opening chapter of this book, the 1980s brought reversal of a long-term trend toward equality of health care in the United States. Under the pressure of rising health care costs in a slow-growth economy, commitments to the disadvantaged gave way to increasing emphasis on personal well-being and material success. Key public decisions altered the financial milieu of the health care system, reducing the subsidies that wealthy and middle-class Americans had given, often unbeknownst, to the poor. This trend signals the ever-increasing importance of personal resources for appropriate care in the event of serious illness. The greatest challenges to public decision-making in the coming years appear to concern the key institution that has historically *lessened* the importance of personal resources in adversity—the welfare state.

It would be a serious error to address the question of cancer survival outside the context of health care as a whole. Although cancer engenders greater fear and attracts more attention than most other diseases, the issues it raises for health care delivery are hardly unique. For everyone, the ready availability of a reliable source of medical care, whose facilities and personnel constitute a familiar part of day-to-day life, would enhance survival chances in all life-threatening diseases. Community-level facilities strictly devoted to cancer detection and treatment appear to have only limited value. The experience of the cancer-detection center described in Chapter 6 illustrates these limitations.

Concern that large numbers of Americans may be losing access to needed health care does not require a compassionate outlook. The middle class itself saw its health care benefits erode in the late twentieth century, incurring liability for more burdensome out-of-pocket payments than had been experienced for generations. In addition, middle-class people found their options as consumers of health care more and more restricted. Fewer and fewer were able to afford insurance that permitted unrestricted selection of physicians. Experts in the 1980s were predicting that nearly everyone would soon be receiving services under a managed-care plan. Researchers have not thus far reported consistent evidence that such plans provide health care very different in quality from traditional settings. But the outcomes of managed care have not received definitive study. The most rigorous studies have focused on Group Health Cooperative, an HMO with important historical distinctions from many of the new health care systems emerging today. Like requirements for out-of-pocket contributions, managed care places restrictions on the patient's range of choice, and these restrictions may unfavorably affect cancer survival or other health care outcomes.

These changes have not altered the ironical contrasts of surfeit and neglect in the health care system. Studies report widespread overtreatment for cancer in the United States. Although American cancer patients in the 1980s did not survive longer than their English counterparts, they were more than five times as likely to receive chemotherapy.[4] Leonard Schaeffer, president of Blue Cross of California, illustrates the impacts of ineffective, desperate cancer treatments on health insurance: "The financial implication of an unscientific 'last ditch' treatment attempt that adds $100,000 to each breast cancer death is staggering. And as the public becomes aware of these treatment fads, it becomes more and more difficult for even responsible physicians to refuse the ineffective treatment to any patient who demands it. In time, the basic financial integrity of the medical plan is jeopardized."[5]

At the same time, there is underinvestment in areas where effective medical interventions are available. As detailed in Chapter 1, health plans in the United States typically cover intensive medical treatment much more richly than checkups for presumably healthy adults, in whom detection of cancer before it produces symptoms may well be life-saving. It is certain that thousands of people die of cancer in the United States every year because they do not receive timely, appropriate, and comparatively inexpensive care.

A national program to ensure decent, basic health care for the disadvantaged may well be the single most effective measure available to improve cancer survival in the United States. A familiar proposal toward this end is that a single, tax-supported health insurance system, covering the needs of all Americans, should be developed. In the atmosphere of concern for the disadvantaged that prevailed in the 1960s and 1970s, liberal politicians proposed concrete programs of this kind. Analysts, however, warned that national health insurance could prove unmanageably expensive. Medicare and Medicaid have opened a floodgate of demand for services and ignited health care hyperinflation. Without severe restrictions on the patient's benefits and options, national health insurance would take the same direction but go infinitely further.

Renewed interest in national health insurance arose from unexpected quarters in the late 1980s. This time, proponents of national health insurance included high-level business executives. Struggling under the burden of providing health insurance for their labor forces, these executives sought an alternative, funded from sources outside their own balance sheets. The new perspective on national health insurance seemed to emphasize funding of services for the employed middle class even more than concern for the disadvantaged.

For the middle class, however, the benefits of national health insurance are uncertain. There are grounds to suspect that such a system would present greater barriers to care and permit less choice than traditional private payment plans have historically offered to the middle class. A national health insurance system would certainly require stringent controls over costs. Reflecting the philosophy of managed care, such controls could restrict the therapeutic options open to cancer patients and the timeliness with which they could obtain a diagnosis or begin treatment. The initiative and intelligent consumer behavior cited above as conducive to individual survival require an atmosphere highly permissive of choice. England and Canada, which both have health care systems predominantly supported by public funds, furnish important examples of tension between the individual's demand for service and the government's efforts to restrain costs. Regulations in both countries strongly discourage provision or consumption of health care outside the system. But every year, thousands of Canadians travel to hospitals in the United States for operations that their provinces lack the capacity to perform. In mid-1991, the British government acknowledged that 700,000 people were on waiting lists for operations, 200,000 having already waited more than a year.[6]

The possibility that a national health insurance system may replace America's current mélange of public and private insurers and providers raises the issue of individual versus collective interests. One important critic has written that health care in the United States has not achieved its potential because it has placed too strong an emphasis on extension of life, even among the desperately ill.[7] In this perspective, resources currently spent on aggressive treatment of an elderly individual with advanced cancer are wasted; they would be better utilized if reallocated to children and expectant mothers for preventive services. This perspective, if incorporated into a national health insurance plan, would almost certainly limit the individual's treatment options. Such a system might deny a gravely ill cancer patient the option of expending personal resources to receive experimental or unorthodox treatment of potential (though perhaps marginal) benefit—a reasonable decision from the individual's point of view.

At this time, establishing a permanent place for health care on the public agenda seems more important than proposing specific solutions. Health care was not a particularly visible public issue in most of the late twentieth century. While the communications media regularly covered the problems of individuals, discussion of system-wide solutions took place only intermittently. Health care did not play a major part in national elections in the United States between the 1970s and the 1990s. Highlighting the importance of resources for health care and their relevance to survival in cancer and other serious diseases will promote an evolutionary sifting of concepts and concrete proposals.

Public discussion of these concepts and proposals will necessarily take place in the context of broader questions regarding the welfare state. Americans tend to react to the term *welfare* with distaste, associating it with gratuitous distribution of benefits to the socially marginal. They sharply distinguish between public assistance for the disadvantaged and programs that protect the middle class from the hazards of modern life: unemployment due to the business cycle; disability due to accident or illness; inability to earn a living due to old age. Many Americans who reject "welfare" support unemployment insurance, disability benefits, and Social Security. While these programs should be considered welfare in a logical sense, they are typically viewed as personally vested benefits, not available to all as rights of citizenship. Given this element of American political culture, it appears unlikely that policymakers will soon promulgate a national health insurance system that will both expand benefits for the disadvantaged and subject the poor and middle class to the same health care standards and restrictions.

A quintessentially American solution to this dilemma would appear to be a dual health insurance system. A system of this kind might provide the disadvantaged with basic care in a highly managed delivery network, yet allow members of the middle class to continue purchasing private health insurance with significant liberty in selection of providers and benefits. Relatively advantaged Americans could attempt to protect themselves against the possibility of major financial liability by utilizing private-sector mechanisms such as high-option health insurance. This approach would be consistent with America's traditional pattern of allowing the coexistence of private and public systems of welfare and social services. In this perspective, the welfare state neither guarantees nor strives for equality. Americans sufficiently advantaged to send their children to private schools still often back the idea of public education. Prominent instigators in the movement to provide Social Security included several with great private fortunes.

The operation of such a system would involve a continuing process of public and private decision-making with respect to the welfare state, which explicitly and implicitly encompasses all payment for health care. Policymakers would continually face the need to decide how generously to fund an insurance program for the poor. Members of the middle class would regularly need to reevaluate the proportion of their earnings to allocate to health insurance versus other needs.

Whatever decisions are made, then, health care will likely remain an area of intense controversy. A dual health insurance system prevailed throughout the late twentieth century. In 1990, all poor Americans were theoretically entitled to care somewhere within the vast complex of public programs from the federal to the county level. Funding of these programs and their successors will make the real difference in availability of care. More important than the formal machinery of the welfare state is the generosity with which it is supported. This proposition holds equally well for the middle class in the funding of its own part of the welfare system. The middle class, for example, will face recurring conflicts over payroll taxation and the scope and choice of services to be covered by Medicare. As with the rest of the welfare state, the debate over health care will encompass conflicts of social values, such as individual versus public interest, immediate consumption versus social saving, and self-funding versus redistribution of resources among both individuals and social classes.

Cancer survival should serve as an index of success or failure of the solutions devised. A system that allocates resources in a manner conducive to the widespread availability of appropriate health care will, all things being equal, promote lower cancer mortality rates over time. Comparisons of trends with those experienced by other advanced industrial countries should prove especially useful. These countries possess the same basic medical technology as the United States but have vastly different systems of delivery and finance. Reflecting economic conditions and public health, the infant mortality rate is often used as an indicator of a society's general well-being. The rate of survival in treatable cancer, which may vary with access to both low- and high-level medical technology, should be used in a similar way.

The Seattle Longitudinal Assessment of Cancer Survival
(SLACS)

Originating as part of a population-based study of pain incidence, the Seattle Longitudinal Assessment of Cancer Survival (SLACS) had the collateral objective of obtaining detailed and comprehensive data on psychological and social factors in cancer mortality. The investigators selected four cancers (lung, pancreatic, prostatic, and cervical) to cover a range of malignancies involving different detection methods, treatment issues, and life expectancies. The study's location—King and Pierce Counties, Washington, where Seattle and Tacoma are located—encompassed a broad range of residential areas, from high-density urban areas to rural-agricultural areas.

Between 1980 and 1982, the investigators collected data on patients twenty through eighty years of age with new diagnoses of the four cancers. The researchers identified these patients through the Cancer Surveillance System (CSS), a population-based tumor registry maintained by the Fred Hutchinson Cancer Research Center in Seattle. Operating under contract with the National Cancer Institute's Surveillance, Epidemiology, and End Results (SEER) Program, the CSS attempts to register all cancer cases occurring in a thirteen-county area in northwest Washington State within three months of diagnosis.

Clinical and demographic information was obtained from the CSS, supplemented by face-to-face interviews with patients and direct communication with physicians when necessary. CSS records provided data on cancer site, stage, and histology, date of diagnosis, gender, location of residence, and source of care. The CSS provided continuing information on patient survival and date of death in the event of mortality.

Face-to-face interviews lasting from two to four hours were conducted for all patients. In the interviews, patients were asked how they became aware that they had cancer. They also were asked about the process of reaching medical care, obtaining a diagnosis, beginning therapy, payments for care, and insurance coverage. The interview schedules included detailed questions on education, occupation, income (personal and family), ethnic background, and family resources. Detailed data on the use of medications for cancer therapy and symptom management were obtained. The interview schedules included several widely used, multi-item indicators to assess the patient's functional level, psychological state, and the impacts of disease. These indicators included the Profile of Mood States (POMS),[1] the Sickness Impact Profile (SIP),[2] and the McGill Pain Questionnaire (MPQ).[3] Instructed to take verbatim notes as well as to administer standardized items, the project interviewers encouraged subjects to comment on the processes of cancer detection, care received, and compliance with regimens.

The investigators monitored the CSS and interviewed patients until prespecified quotas for each malignancy were filled. A total of 877 living individuals with the four malignancies specified above were identified during an eighteen-month accrual period. Ethical considerations required that investigators obtain permission from each potential subject's physician before requesting an interview. Permission was obtained for contacting 599 of these patients, of whom 536 agreed to interviews and provided sufficient data to be included in the analysis. Of those interviewed, 201 had prostatic cancer; 260, lung cancer; 25, cancer of the pancreas; and 50, cancer of the cervix. These patients were followed through the CSS to update vital status until mid-1987. Patients for whom no record of death appeared in the registry were followed for up to eighty months from date of diagnosis. All were followed for at least five years.

The researchers carried out several procedures to estimate bias in the sample of cancer patients obtained and assess its potential effect on substantive findings. In the first procedure, they asked physicians who withheld permission to contact specific patients for their reasons for refusal. The physicians predominantly cited reasons of extreme morbidity among the patients, including emotional problems, compromised mental functioning, and moribund status. Second, at the midpoint of the study, the investigators compared the patients they had succeeded in interviewing with the names entered in the CSS over the same time period. Those interviewed were more likely to have received surgical treatment than those not interviewed. No differences were detected in age, race, and marital status. Finally, the investigators compared the 201 prostate cancer patients interviewed with 1,000 consecutive prostate cancer patients entered in the CSS during an overlapping time period. The interviewed patients tended to be younger (mean age: interviewed = 67.6; not interviewed = 68.8; $p < .05$), diagnosed at a higher stage (mean stage: interviewed = 1.8; not interviewed = 1.5; $p < .01$), and more likely to be HMO members (percentage in HMO: interviewed = 20.7; not interviewed = 6.5; $p < .01$). Although patients with extreme morbidity and debilitation (diagnosed with all four malignancies) seemed relatively unlikely to have entered the study, no consistent evidence appeared to indicate that those interviewed differed in other respects from the populations from which they were drawn.

While no consistent evidence was obtained to suggest that those interviewed differed markedly from those not interviewed, it is safest to view the 536 patients in the SLACS as representing no definite population. However, relationships among variables of primary interest seemed similar when computed on the basis of the SLACS sample and the population of cancer patients from which it was drawn. Logistic regression and Cox proportional hazards models predicting care received and mortality risk among prostate cancer patients were highly similar when based on either the 201 patients interviewed in the SLACS or the 1,000 consecutive patients selected from the CSS.

The CSS constitutes a highly reliable means of identifying cancer patients and monitoring their survival. An evaluation of the CSS has recently demonstrated that fewer than 2.5 percent of the cancer cases in its catchment area are missed by the registry.[4] Several methods are used to ensure complete and timely inclusion of mortality data on all patients. The National Cancer Institute requires the registry to update the status of all living patients within a maximum of eighteen months following diagnosis or last contact.[5] The CSS accomplishes this update, first, by contacting the hospitals at which patients were originally treated and the physicians who cared for them.[6] Death certificates are used as an additional means of follow-up,[7] the names of all those in the registry being compared with a computerized file in the state capital. Periodic monitoring and audit procedures are conducted by the National Cancer Institute.

Data from the CSS records and the patient interviews were merged into a single data set, which was supplemented with census tract data from the 1980 U.S. Census. Major data elements and their sources are specified in Table A-1.

Table A-1 *Major Elements in the SLACS Data Base:*
Sources and Applications in Models of Mortality

	Data Element	Source	Application
A. Outcome Variables	1. Vital status[a]	CSS	Compute dependent variables (five-year survival and follow-up time)
	2. Date of death[a]	CSS	
B. Intermediate Factors	1. Treatment(s) received[b] a. surgery b. radiation c. chemotherapy	CSS and Interview	Intervening variables (observed and computed)
	2. Date of diagnosis[c]	CSS and Interview	
	3. Date, beginning of treatment[c]		
	4. Date, first suspicion of illness[c]	Interview	
	5. Pain at diagnosis	Interview	
	6. Detection of cancer at routine physical	Interview	
	7. Stage	CSS	
C. Independent Variables	1. Income (family, year preceding cancer diagnosis)	Interview	Test SES hypotheses
	2. Education (years completed)	Interview	Test SES hypotheses
	3. Occupation[d] a. self (recent) b. self (usual) c. spouse (recent) d. spouse (usual)	Interview	Test SES hypotheses
	4. Wealth	1980 Census (imputed)	Test SES hypotheses
	5. Profile of mood states	Interview	Test emotional hypothesis
	6. Sickness impact profile		Test emotional hypothesis

	Data Element	Source	Application
	7. HMO membership	CSS	Test HMO hypothesis
D. Background Information	1. Sex	CSS	Control variables, all hypotheses
	2. Age	CSS	
	3. Race	CSS	
	4. Marital status	CSS	
	5. Disease site	CSS	
	6. Histology	CSS	
	7. Ethnicity	Interview	
	8. Copayment	Interview	

[a]"Vital status," a dummy variable indicating whether the patient was alive or dead in any given month after diagnosis, and date of death (if the patient had died) are used jointly to compute five-year survival. They are also used jointly to determine the number of months the patient was followed after diagnosis until death for the purpose of computing mortality risk over the entire follow-up period. If no death date was recorded in the CSS, a follow-up time of 80 months from the beginning of the study was assumed.

[b]As well as indicating individual treatments the patient has received, this variable is used to compute receipt of multimodal therapy (combining two or more modalities), an indication of "intensity of care."

[c]Date of diagnosis is used to compute two indices of delay: lag time between date of diagnosis and the beginning of treatment, possibly a "system-initiated" form of delay; and lag between the time the patient first suspected he or she was ill and date of diagnosis, a form of delay more closely related to patient behavior.

[d]For each occupation reported, occupational prestige is computed on the basis of the widely used scale developed by O. D. Duncan and P. M. Blau (*The American Occupational Structure* [New York: Wiley, 1967]).

APPENDIX B

Statistical Methods and Tables

General

Statistical analysis aimed at estimating the effects of mood states, early-detection processes, socioeconomic status, and HMO membership on care received and survival, after adjusting for the effects of personal-background variables and disease characteristics. Selection of right-hand variables for these models differed according to expectations of determinants of the dependent variable based on the literature of health behavior—for example, the Behavioral Model of Health Services Utilization.[1] Ordinary least squares multiple regression was used to model continuous dependent variables—namely, stage when diagnosed and months from diagnosis to treatment. Logistic multiple regression was used to model dichotomous dependent variables, such as cancer detection at a routine physical and multimodal treatment. The Cox proportional hazards model was used to estimate relative mortality risk. The investigators used the Statistical Analysis System (SAS) to perform all statistical procedures.

Figures 5 through 8 (Chapters 5 through 8) present model-based five-year survival rates across categories of cancer patients. These figures are intended to promote rapid comprehension of the major findings reported in this book among readers unfamiliar with the basic analytical techniques of biostatistics, econometrics, or health services research.

214

Represented as a dichotomous dependent variable, five-year survival is modeled on the basis of logistic multiple regression equations. Estimation of coefficients in equations reflecting this model (fitting the model to observed data via maximum likelihood) permits computation of percentages in each category of patients (e.g., high versus low socioeconomic status), adjusted for the influence of background variables (such as age and cancer stage). Thus, the percentages of five-year survivors presented are estimates of percentages for hypothetical groups of individuals with identical characteristics in all respects (mean values on all background variables) except the subject of comparison in the figure.

In the model, the probability of an individual's surviving five years, p, is expressed as:

$$\text{Log}\,[p/(1 - p)] = b_0 + b_1 X_1 + b_2 X_2 + \ldots + b_k X_k$$

The values $X_1 \ldots X_k$ describe characteristics of an individual patient, such as age, sex, and stage. The b's are coefficients that reflect the influence of these characteristics on the probability p. The standard error of each coefficient is determined in the fitting process. Using the standard error, investigators can test a coefficient to determine whether it is significantly different from zero, a value that indicates no influence of a variable on the five-year survival rate. Once the logistic regression model has been fit, percentages are calculated as $100 \times p$.

The investigators estimated relative mortality risk by using stratified and unstratified versions of the Cox proportional hazards model.[2] In this model, the probability of death in any time period over the length of the study—t_j for an individual who has survived to the beginning of that period [the individual's "hazard rate" in that time period, denoted $H(t_j)$]—is equal to a "baseline" probability of death in that time period for the sample as a whole, $H_0(t_j)$, multiplied by a time-invariant function of the individual's characteristics. Specifically, for an individual with characteristics $(X_1 \ldots X_k)$, the model specifies the following relationship:

$$H(t) = H_0(t)\,exp(b_1 X_1 + \ldots + b_k X_k)$$

This model is constructed so that the relative risk of death due to a one-unit positive difference in the value of X_k, with all other characteristics unchanged, is simply $exp(b_k)$. Maximum likelihood estimates for the coefficients $(b_1 \ldots b_k)$ were calculated by means of the procedure PHGLM of the Statistical Analysis System.[3]

Applying this model separately to each disease site sometimes necessitated making estimates on the basis of very small numbers of observations in some cells. As an alternative, the investigators developed an aggregate model combining several cancer sites. The stratified version of the Cox proportional hazards model permits estimation of a single equation, which indicates the effects of variables of interest while taking account of differences in mortality patterns among diseases. This stratified model computes baseline mortality probabilities separately by disease, so that, instead of a single $H_0(t)$ as in the above equation, estimation takes place on the basis of $H_{0i}(t)$, where $i = 1, 2, 3, 4$ indexes separate disease sites.[4] The use of baseline hazard rates specific to each cancer permits the aggregation of diseases of different sites, which may have different mortality patterns but in which individual characteristics affect mortality in the same way.

Analyses supporting Chapters 5 through 8 include models based on combined cancer sites, such as the stratified Cox proportional hazards model, and models based on individual sites. Findings based only on combined sites are presented in the figures and tables for Chapter 5. Both combined and disease-specific estimates are presented in the figures and tables for Chapters 6 through 8.

Chapter 5:
Emotional Health and Cancer Survival

In assessing the relationship between psychological factors and cancer survival, the investigators made two assumptions. First, if emotional factors affect survival, they should have a similar effect among people with all types of cancer. Second, the emotional characteristics of cancer patients should be invariant across place of residence, educational level, and family income. Consistent with these assumptions, right-hand variables in associated models include only estimates of psychological factors and basic individual background and illness-related variables (such as disease site and stage).

In the data analysis, three categories of "psychological disturbance" were identified within each POMS subscale and the SIP Emotional

Behavior scale. Individuals scoring approximately in the top 20 percent of numerical values obtained on each subscale were considered to have "extreme" symptoms on the corresponding dimension. Those scoring below the top 20 percent but above the lowest 40 percent were considered to have "slight" symptoms. Those scoring within the lowest 40 percent were not considered to be disturbed along the pertinent dimension: with respect to tension, depression, etc., their symptoms were characterized as "none."

Statistical analysis compared persons in the "slight" and "extreme" categories with those in the "none" category. Two sets of multivariate models were estimated. Both included dummy variables on the right-hand side indicating slight and extreme disturbance. Coefficients estimated for these dummy variables indicated differences between each category of emotional disturbance and a category omitted from the equations: no disturbance ("none") according to the specified dimension.

The first set of equations predicted five-year survival as a dichotomous variable. These equations were logistic multiple regressions. Based on all four cancer sites, each equation included three dummy variables on the right-hand side representing pancreatic, prostatic, and cervical; coefficients on these variables reflected differences from lung cancer (omitted from the equations) on the outcome variable. Coefficients from these equations are presented in Table B-5.1 and serve as the basis for Figure 5 in Chapter 5.

A second set of equations was estimated in order to model relative mortality hazard for individuals in each category of psychological disturbance. These equations are Cox proportional hazards models. Table B-5.2 summarizes results of this analysis. Separate models are estimated for each dimension of the POMS, a single subscale of the POMS being represented in each equation. The equations indicate statistically significant findings on the POMS dimensions of Confusion, Fatigue, and Vigor, but not on Tension, Depression, or Anger.

Only models based on all four cancers combined are presented here; presenting all possible models would have necessitated reproduction of forty-eight equations. Models run on each individual cancer, however, yielded results generally duplicative of those shown here.

Table B-5.1 Profile of Mood States (POMS) Dimensions Predicting Five-Year Survival: Logistic Regression (Standard Errors in Parentheses)

POMS Dimension					
A. Tension					
Slight	.240 (.328)	—	—	—	—
Extreme	-.100 (.292)	—	—	—	—
B. Depression					
Slight	.133 (.297)	—	—	—	—
Extreme	-.149 (.305)	—	—	—	—
C. Anger					
Slight	-.148 (.299)	—	—	—	—
Extreme	.351 (.310)	—	—	—	—
D. Confusion					
Slight	-.235 (.284)	—	—	—	—
Extreme	-.351 (.296)	—	—	—	—
E. Fatigue					
Slight	-.697* (.326)	—	—	—	—

Extreme	—	—	—	—	-.617* (.298)	—
F. Vigor						
Slight	—	—	—	—	—	.430 (.296)
Extreme	—	—	—	—	—	.262 (.294)
Patient Characteristic						
Sex	.488 (.335)	.467 (.334)	.482 (.336)	.459 (.335)	.461 (.337)	.467 (.336)
Age	-.023 (.013)	-.024 (.012)	-.020 (.013)	-.024 (.013)	-.027* (.013)	-.022 (.012)
Cancer Stage	-1.233** (.151)	-1.235** (.152)	-1.250** (.153)	-1.233** (.152)	-1.247** (.153)	-1.250** (.152)
Cancer Site						
Pancreas	-.391 (.679)	-.316 (.675)	-.368 (.675)	-.322 (.676)	-.231 (.675)	-.393 (.676)
Prostate	2.086** (.317)	2.094** (.317)	2.055** (.318)	2.064** (.317)	2.053** (.321)	2.020** (.324)
Cervix	.954 (.492)	.961 (.491)	.985* (.495)	.936 (.491)	.833 (.494)	.880 (.487)

$*p < .05$
$**p < .01$

Table B-5.2 *Profile of Mood States (POMS) Dimensions and Relative Mortality Risk: Proportional Hazards Models*

	B Coeff.	Risk Ratio	Std. Error	Confidence Limits Lower	Upper	p Value
A. Tension						
Tension Level						
Slight	−.081	.922	.174	.653	1.302	.64
Extreme	.079	1.082	.152	.801	1.462	.60
Sex	−.402	.669	.157	.490	.913	<.02
Age	.007	1.007	.007	.994	1.020	.31
Cancer Stage	.804	2.234	.083	1.896	2.634	<.01
B. Depression						
Depression Level						
Slight	−.094	.910	.161	.662	1.252	.56
Extreme	.128	1.137	.158	.831	1.554	.42
Sex	−.388	.678	.158	.496	.928	<.02
Age	.008	1.008	.007	.994	1.022	.25
Cancer Stage	.796	2.217	.087	1.866	2.633	<.01
C. Anger						
Anger Level						
Slight	.023	1.023	.153	.756	1.385	.88
Extreme	−.051	.950	.170	.679	1.331	.76
Sex	−.382	.682	.156	.501	.929	<.02
Age	.006	1.006	.007	.992	1.020	.35
Cancer Stage	.804	2.234	.084	1.892	2.639	<.01
D. Confusion						
Confusion Level						
Slight	.366	1.442	.150	1.071	1.941	<.02
Extreme	.163	1.177	.154	.868	1.597	.29
Sex	−.399	.671	.156	.493	.914	<.02
Age	.006	1.006	.007	.992	1.020	.36
Cancer Stage	.809	2.246	.083	1.905	2.647	<.01
E. Fatigue						
Fatigue Level						
Slight	.310	1.363	.164	.985	1.887	.06
Extreme	.357	1.429	.151	1.060	1.927	<.02
Sex	−.406	.666	.157	.488	.909	<.01
Age	.008	1.008	.007	.994	1.022	.25
Cancer Stage	.794	2.212	.083	1.877	2.607	<.01

	B Coeff.	Risk Ratio	Std. Error	Confidence Limits		p Value
				Lower	Upper	
F. Vigor						
Vigor Level						
Slight	−.506	.603	.165	.435	.836	<.01
Extreme	−.338	.713	.180	.499	1.019	.06
Sex	−.436	.647	.157	.474	.882	<.01
Age	.004	1.004	.007	.990	1.018	.54
Cancer Stage	.841	2.319	.085	1.960	2.744	<.01

Chapter 6: Early Detection?

Chapter 6 identifies four independent variables conceptually associated with early detection of cancer, and it uses these variables in statistical models to predict (1) stage at diagnosis and (2) survival. Stage, a classification of degree of dissemination of a malignancy at the time of diagnosis, is used as an intervening variable in the data analysis, in part to help assess the importance of lead-time bias in the study reported here. Data for the analysis include three of the malignancies covered by the SLACS: lung, prostatic, and cervical. Because of the very high mortality in pancreatic cancer and the small likelihood that early detection (and most other interventions) would improve survival, this disease site is omitted from analysis here and in all subsequent chapters.

The four variables reflecting alternative dimensions of early detection include (1) time elapsed from first suspicion of illness to date of diagnosis; (2) detection at a routine physical examination; (3) absence versus presence of pain at the time the cancer was detected; (4) time elapsed from diagnosis until the beginning of the first course of treatment. Values on these variables were determined on the basis of data from patient interviews and from the CSS tumor registry records maintained by the Fred Hutchinson Cancer Research Center. On occasion, project personnel contacted physicians' offices directly to obtain information missing from the registry.

Specifically, values on these four variables were computed as follows:

1. *Time from first suspicion of illness to diagnosis.* The patient's malignancy was referenced in the interviews in language initiated by the subject to describe his or her "health problem." An interview item asked the subject, "When did you first suspect you had this problem?" The value on this variable was the time elapsed between the date so identified and the date recorded in the registry of the beginning of the first course of treatment.

2. *Detection at a routine physical examination.* Interviewers were instructed to utilize verbal probes to encourage subjects to indicate how their illnesses were detected. The most frequent responses identified pain, bleeding, or some other symptom that aroused the subject's suspicion of cancer; less frequently, the subject indicated that he or she had seen a physician for symptoms that did not arouse suspicion of cancer but turned out to be associated with a malignancy; others visited physicians for conditions unrelated to cancer and had their malignancies detected incidentally. A minority (about one-third) gave none of these responses, indicating that they had had their cancers detected at a routine physical and had not suspected they had cancer or any other disease before that time.

3. *Absence of pain at detection.* Following the item asking when the patient first suspected he or she was ill, the interview schedule contained an item asking whether pain was present at that time. It was assumed that such pain would have remained until actual diagnosis.

4. *Time from diagnosis to treatment.* This variable was computed on the basis of tumor registry data, which included the date of diagnosis according to pathology reports and date of the beginning of the first course of treatment according to physicians' offices. In the analysis, lag periods were computed on the basis of the months in which diagnosis and the beginning of treatment occurred.

Stage, an important variable in this analysis, helps to distinguish degrees of effectiveness for different aspects of the detection process and to assess the importance of lead-time bias. The CSS included cancer stage, determined on the basis of a standard classification scheme for each disease.[5] Stage was considered as a continuous variable with three degrees.

Tables B-6.1 through B-6.5 represent the detailed analysis referenced in the body of Chapter 6, including multivariate analyses of various kinds. All these tables present separate analyses for (1) all disease sites combined and (2) each individual disease.

Table B-6.1 presents coefficients from ordinary least squares regression equations predicting cancer stage. Independent variables correspond to the four dimensions of early detection specified above. These equations all include age, and, where appropriate, sex, on the right-hand side. The equation for all malignancies combined includes dummy variables representing prostatic and cervical cancer. Coefficients on these variables represent differences between the individual malignancies and lung cancer.

Table B-6.1 *Early-Detection Variables and Cancer Stage: Regression Coefficients (Standard Errors in Parentheses)*

A. All Sites

Early-Detection Variable

Suspicion to Diagnosis (months)	−.022 (.013)	—	—	—
Detected at Physical	—	−.342** (.095)	—	—
No Pain at Detection	—	—	−.345** (.091)	—
Diagnosis to Treatment (months)	—	—	—	−.012 (.048)

Patient Characteristic

Sex	−.129 (.123)	−.088 (.122)	−.103 (.121)	−.133 (.123)
Age	.003 (.005)	.003 (.005)	.006 (.005)	.003 (.005)

Cancer Site

Prostate	−.426** (.112)	−.414** (.109)	−.425** (.109)	−.447** (.113)
Cervix	−.591** (.177)	−.590** (.174)	−.510** (.175)	−.588** (.180)
$R^2 =$	.11	.14	.15	.11

B. Lung

Early-Detection Variable

Suspicion to Diagnosis (months)	−.042 (.028)	—	—	—
Detected at Physical	—	−.315* (.133)	—	—
No Pain at Detection	—	—	−.149 (.123)	—
Diagnosis to Treatment (months)	—	—	—	.136 (.095)

Patient Characteristic

Sex	−.129 (.119)	−.088 (.119)	.117 (.119)	−.103 (.120)
Age	.002 (.006)	.006 (.006)	.006 (.007)	.004 (.006)
$R^2 =$	.02	.04	.02	.02

Continued on next page

Table B-6.1 *Continued*

C. Prostate

Early-Detection
Variable

Suspicion to Diagnosis (months)	−.015 (.009)	—	—	—
Detected at Physical	—	−.353* (.173)	—	—
No Pain at Detection	—	—	−.604** (.165)	—
Diagnosis to Treatment (months)	—	—	—	−.049 (.077)

Patient Characteristic

Age	−.004 (.010)	−.013 (.011)	.007 (.010)	−.009 (.011)
$R^2 =$	.02	.04	.12	.01

D. Cervix

Early-Detection
Variable

Suspicion to Diagnosis (months)	.102** (.031)	—	—	—
Detected at Physical	—	−.546** (.185)	—	—
No Pain at Detection	—	—	−.438* (.215)	—
Diagnosis to Treatment (months)	—	—	—	−.044 (.066)

Patient Characteristic

Age	.014 (.006)	.013 (.007)	.013 (.007)	.014 (.008)
$R^2 =$	.31	.26	.18	.09

*$p < .05$
**$p < .01$

Table B-6.2 *Early-Detection Variables and Five-Year Survival:*
Logistic Regression (Standard Errors in Parentheses)

A. All Sites

Early-Detection
Variable

Suspicion to Diagnosis Two Months or More	−.380 (.251)	—	—	—
Detected at Physical	—	1.076** (.226)	—	—
No Pain at Detection	—	—	.855** (.219)	—
Diagnosis to Treatment Two Months or More	—	—	—	−.158 (.311)

Patient Characteristic

Sex	.624* (.304)	.535 (.310)	.572 (.307)	.607* (.304)
Age	−.026* (.011)	−.026* (.011)	−.030** (.011)	−.026* (.011)

Cancer Site

Prostate	2.333** (.279)	2.279** (.284)	2.303** (.281)	2.322** (.281)
Cervix	1.258** (.415)	1.240** (.424)	1.084** (.419)	1.234** (.414)

B. Lung

Early-Detection
Variable

Suspicion to Diagnosis Two Months or More	−.152 (.401)	—	—	—
Detected at Physical	—	1.145** (.332)	—	—
No Pain at Detection	—	—	.182 (.320)	—
Diagnosis to Treatment Two Months or More	—	—	—	−7.350 (21.137)

Patient Characteristic

Sex	.619* (.304)	.539 (.312)	−.030 (.016)	.560 (.306)
Age	−.028 (.016)	−.037* (.017)	.603* (.304)	−.029 (.158)

Continued on next page

Table B-6.2 *Continued*

C. Prostate

Early-Detection
Variable

Suspicion to Diagnosis Two Months or More	−.206 (.363)	—	—	—
Detected at Physical	—	.940** (.343)	—	—
No Pain at Detection	—	—	1.357** (.321)	—
Diagnosis to Treatment Two Months or More	—	—	—	.180 (.387)

Patient Characteristic

Age	−.011 (.021)	−.002 (.021)	−.007 (.021)	−.009 (.020)

D. Cervix

Early-Detection
Variable

Suspicion to Diagnosis Two Months or More	−1.498* (.691)	—	—	—
Detected at Physical	—	1.775* (.845)	—	—
No Pain at Detection	—	—	1.728* (.746)	—
Diagnosis to Treatment Two Months or More	—	—	—	−.378 (.824)

Patient Characteristic

Age	−.049 (.026)	−.037 (.025)	−.049 (.026)	−.042 (.025)

*$p < .05$
**$p < .01$

Table B-6.3 *Early-Detection Variables and Relative Mortality Risk: Proportional Hazards Models*

Part I. Independent Variable: Detected at Routine Physical

	B Coeff.	Risk Ratio	Std. Error	Confidence Limits Lower	Upper	p Value
A. All Sites						
Routine Phys.	−.743	.476	.149	.354	.639	<.01
Sex	−.288	.750	.147	.560	1.003	.05
Age	.012	1.012	.007	.988	1.036	.06
B. Lung						
Routine Phys.	−.637	.529	.182	.369	.759	<.01
Sex	−.302	.739	.148	.551	.992	<.05
Age	.010	1.010	.008	.995	1.026	.17
C. Prostate						
Routine Phys.	−.770	.463	.272	.270	.793	<.01
Age	.009	1.009	.017	.977	1.043	.58
D. Cervix						
Routine Phys.	−8.739	.000	30.0406	N.A.[a]	N.A.	.77
Age	.021	1.021	.021	.980	1.064	.32

[a]Not Applicable. Confidence limits too large for column limitations because of large standard error

Part II. Independent Variable: No Pain at Detection

	B Coeff.	Risk Ratio	Std. Error	Confidence Limits Lower	Upper	p Value
A. All Sites						
No Pain	−.454	.635	.123	.498	.811	<.01
Sex	−.341	.711	.147	.531	.952	<.05
Age	.015	1.015	.007	1.002	1.029	<.05
B. Lung						
No Pain	−.193	.824	.152	.610	1.113	.20
Sex	−.369	.692	.148	.516	.926	<.05
Age	.010	1.010	.008	.994	1.026	.22
C. Prostate						
No Pain	−.913	.401	.231	.254	.634	<.01
Age	.008	1.008	.016	.976	1.041	.63
D. Cervix						
No Pain	−1.604	.201	.598	.062	.657	<.01
Age	.048	1.049	.024	1.000	1.100	<.05

Table B-6.4 *Early-Detection Variables and Five-Year Survival:*
Logistic Regression Analysis, Including Stage
(Standard Errors in Parentheses)

A. All Sites

Early-Detection
Variable

Suspicion to Diagnosis Two Months or More	−.507 (.288)	—	—	—
Detected at Physical	—	.888** (.262)	—	—
No Pain at Detection	—	—	.338 (.251)	—
Diagnosis to Treatment Two Months or More	—	—	—	−.104 (.383)

Patient
Characteristic

Sex	.496 (.342)	.430 (.345)	.484 (.339)	.486 (.340)
Age	−.020 (.012)	−.019 (.013)	−.019 (.012)	−.017 (.012)

Cancer Site

Prostate	2.043** (.315)	1.977** (.317)	1.990** (.313)	2.013** (.316)
Cervix	.799 (.469)	.791 (.475)	.683 (.467)	.759 (.464)
Cancer Stage	−1.206** (.151)	−1.116** (.152)	−1.155** (.153)	−1.200** (.150)

B. Lung

Early-Detection
Variable

Suspicion to Diagnosis Two Months or More	−.053 (.436)	—	—	—
Detected at Physical	—	.958* (.378)	—	—
No Pain at Detection	—	—	.044 (.358)	—

Diagnosis to Treatment Two Months or More	—	—	—	−8.177 N.A.
Patient Characteristic				
Sex	.484 (.342)	.419 (.350)	.482 (.342)	.439 (.345)
Age	−.001 (.018)	−.017 (.018)	−.010 (.018)	−.012 (.018)
Cancer Stage	−1.225** (.247)	−1.146** (.249)	−1.225** (.247)	−1.225** (.251)
C. Prostate				
Early-Detection Variable				
Suspicion to Diagnosis Two Months or More	−.514 (.423)	—	—	—
Detected at Physical	—	.624 (.395)	—	—
No Pain at Detection	—	—	.519 (.390)	—
Diagnosis to Treatment Two Months or More	—	—	—	.501 (.490)
Patient Characteristic				
Age	−.015 (.024)	−.007 (.024)	−.010 (.024)	−.011 (.024)
Cancer Stage	−1.140** (.200)	−1.056** (.201)	−1.013** (.210)	−1.114** (.198)
D. Cervix				
Early-Detection Variable				
Suspicion to Diagnosis Two Months or More	−1.964* (.900)	—	—	—

Continued on next page

Table B-6.4 *Continued*

Detected at Physical	—	1.936 (1.154)	—	—
No Pain at Detection	—	—	1.475 (.923)	—
Diagnosis to Treatment Two Months or More	—	—	—	−1.349 (1.071)
Patient Characteristic				
Age	−.055 (.033)	−.042 (.030)	−.047 (.030)	−.049 (.031)
Cancer Stage	−1.898* (.796)	−1.326 (.702)	−1.774* (.788)	−2.000** (.763)

*$p < .05$
**$p < .01$

Table B-6.5 *Early-Detection Variables and Relative Mortality Risk: Proportional Hazards Models, Including Stage*

Part I. Independent Variable: Detected at Routine Physical

	B Coeff.	Risk Ratio	Std. Error	Confidence Limits Lower	Confidence Limits Upper	p Value
A. All Sites						
Routine Phys.	−.607	.545	.167	.392	.758	<.01
Sex	−.343	.709	.163	.513	.980	<.05
Age	.004	1.004	.007	.990	1.018	.56
Cancer Stage	.775	2.171	.085	1.834	2.571	<.01
B. Lung						
Routine Phys.	−.579	.560	.209	.371	.847	<.01
Sex	−.344	.709	.164	.513	.981	<.05
Age	.001	1.001	.008	.985	1.018	.87
Cancer Stage	.677	1.968	.111	1.581	2.451	<.01
C. Prostate						
Routine Phys.	−.453	.636	.286	.361	1.120	.11
Age	.000	1.000	.016	.969	1.032	.99
Cancer Stage	.861	2.364	.140	1.793	3.119	<.01
D. Cervix						
Routine Phys.	−8.174	.000	31.515	N.A.	N.A.	.79
Age	.016	1.016	.025	.968	1.067	.52
Cancer Stage	1.322	3.752	.450	1.539	9.150	<.01

Part II. Independent Variable: No Pain at Detection

	B Coeff.	Risk Ratio	Std. Error	Confidence Limits Lower	Confidence Limits Upper	p Value
A. All Sites						
No Pain	−.213	.808	.135	.619	1.056	.12
Sex	−.384	.681	.164	.493	.942	<.02
Age	.005	1.005	.007	.991	1.020	.49
Cancer Stage	.799	2.223	.085	1.877	2.633	<.01
B. Lung						
No Pain	−.110	.896	.167	.643	1.248	.51
Sex	−.392	.676	.164	.489	.934	<.02
Age	.000	1.000	.009	.982	1.017	.97
Cancer Stage	.704	2.022	.109	1.629	2.509	<.01

Continued on next page

Table B-6.5 *Continued*

	B Coeff.	Risk Ratio	Std. Error	Confidence Limits		*p* Value
				Lower	*Upper*	
C. Prostate						
No Pain	−.255	.775	.261	.463	1.299	.32
Age	.000	1.000	.016	.969	1.033	.98
Cancer Stage	.859	2.361	.148	1.762	3.164	<.01
D. Cervix						
No Pain	−.615	.540	.768	.118	2.471	.42
Age	.029	1.029	.027	.976	1.086	.28
Cancer Stage	1.363	3.906	.507	1.433	10.648	<.01

Table B-6.1 presents consistent evidence that (1) detection at a routine physical examination and (2) diagnosis in the absence of pain predict lower disease stage. The coefficient on time from first suspicion to diagnosis predicts stage at a statistically significant level only for cancer of the cervix. No statistically significant results were found for time from diagnosis to treatment.

Table B-6.2 presents results of a logistic regression analysis of five-year survival computed as a dichotomous variable. Right-hand variables in the equations are the same as those in Table B-6.1. Time from suspicion to diagnosis and from diagnosis to treatment, continuous variables as observed, are represented as dichotomous variables. Predicted percentages of five-year survival presented in Figure 6 in the body of Chapter 6 are computed from the logistic regression coefficients.

The pattern of statistically significant relations in Table B-6.2 is similar to that observed in Table B-6.1, detection at a routine physical and absence of pain at time of diagnosis predicting greater five-year survival in nearly all instances. Time from suspicion to diagnosis is a statistically significant predictor only for cervical cancer, with greater elapsed time predicting reduced survival.

For the two early-detection variables of greatest interest, Table B-6.3 presents coefficients from Cox proportional hazards models. Because a version of the model stratified by disease site was used in the equation combining all disease sites, no dummy variables representing individual disease sites were included. The pattern of statistically significant relations in Table B-6.3 is highly similar to that in Table B-6.2. A similar Cox equation had the following coefficients for time (months) from suspicion to diagnosis: all three cancers combined, $-.003$ (s.e. = .015); lung, $-.014$ (s.e. = .036); prostate, $-.012$ (s.e. = .021); cervix, .422 (s.e. = .103). A similar equation had the following coefficients for time (months) from diagnosis to treatment: all three cancers combined, .086 (s.e. = .066); lung, .356 (s.e. = .124); prostate, $-.109$ (s.e. = .112); cervix, .184 (s.e. = .133).

It should be noted that confidence limits are not presented in Table B-6.3 (Part I) for the risk ratio on detection at a routine physical in cervical cancer. The standard error on the coefficient was large and thus generated extremely high confidence limits for the risk ratios, requiring more space than column limitations in the table permitted. Thus, the lower and upper confidence limits are designated as not applicable (N.A.). This limitation has been noted for cervical cancer in several other tables. Readers should take appropriate caution in interpreting findings for cervical cancer where this note appears.

Table B-6.4 presents a logistic analysis similar to that in Table B-6.2, except that stage has been added to the right-hand side of the equations. With the addition of stage, nearly all relations between detection at a routine physical, absence of pain at detection (right-hand variables), and five-year survival fail to achieve the .05 level of significance. This observation supports the assumption that stage is an intervening variable between these dimensions of early detection and five-year survival. A relation between detection at a routine physical and five-year survival remains statistically significant only for lung cancer.

Table B-6.5 presents Cox proportional hazards models similar to those in Table B-6.4. The same results of adding stage to the survival models as occurred in Table B-6.4 occur in Table B-6.5.

Two additional Cox equations were estimated for lung cancer patients aged sixty-five and under, diagnosed in Stage I or II, and with non–small cell disease. Results here were more similar to those obtained for prostate and cervical cancer. In an equation including the right-hand variables sex and age, detection at a routine physical significantly predicted mortality risk (B coefficient = $-.844$, s.e. = .352). When stage was added to the equation, this coefficient became $-.693$ (s.e. = .374), no longer significant at the $p < .05$ level.

Evidence that stage functions as an intervening variable between early detection and survival is, in turn, evidence that the observed survival gains are substantive—that is, not merely the reflection of lead-time bias. If the observed relationships between indices of early detection (detection at a routine physical and in the absence of pain) and survival merely reflect lead-time bias, these relationships should be observable within key segments of the natural history of the disease. Including stage in the logistic and Cox equations effectively results in a within-stage analysis of survival. The fact that these relationships are reduced in magnitude and no longer statistically significant in this analysis suggests that the observation of increased survival time cannot be interpreted as merely having watched the patient longer.

Chapter 7: Class and Cancer Survival

To assess the relation between socioeconomic status and cancer survival, this chapter focused on two of the most readily measurable dimensions of social stratification: income and education. The degree to which these dimensions subsume the concept of socioeconomic status is, of course, open to dispute. But it is the consensus of American social scientists that these two variables constitute the principal dimensions of social differentiation operative in the United States in the late twentieth century. These variables have the added advantage of being measurable, capable of being assessed through questionnaire items used in survey research.

This basic analytical framework admits additional and related dimensions of socioeconomic status. "Occupational prestige" frequently concerns sociologists, who have developed scales to determine the degree of esteem the American public grants each occupation. This dimension seems likely to capture both income and education, both of which would presumably rise with higher occupational status. Economists have identified "wealth" as more important than income. In this connection, wealth includes savings, capital investments, and personal property, such as real estate. As a means of acquiring goods and services that are especially costly or needed in emergencies, wealth may be more important than income. A person with significant wealth yet relatively low income may, for example, be better able to finance a course of intensive medical treatment than one with high income and little wealth. The former could draw upon assets to generate large amounts of cash; the latter might be limited to his or her level of current income.

The SLACS researchers collected data on all these dimensions of socioeconomic status. The questionnaire used in the face-to-face interviews included items on income, education, and occupation. The item on income aimed at determining family income, requesting the subject to indicate how much all those in the household received from all sources. Subjects were asked to indicate their household-income levels in $5,000 increments from "under $5,000" to "$60,000 and over." To determine educational level, the interview schedule included an item asking how many years of schooling the subject completed. To determine occupation, the interview schedule included an item asking subjects to indicate the occupation in which they had been employed the longest over their entire career. A score was determined for the occupation named according to the widely used scale developed by Duncan and Blau.[6] Female subjects were asked to name their husbands' "usual" occupation as well; these subjects received their husbands' occupational prestige score if it exceeded their own. The researchers used census tract data on home values as an index of wealth. On the pertinent variable, each subject received a score equal to the median value reported by the 1980 U.S. Census of the homes in the tract where he or she resided.

As a preliminary step in the analysis, the researchers examined these four variables to assess the best combination to be used in building models and methods for combining them to increase power and efficiency. First, the researchers performed a principal components analysis to assess the analytical strength that might be added by constructing a socioeconomic-status scale using two or more of these variables and weighing each variable differentially. The principal components analysis, however, did not suggest a differential weighing scheme (coefficients of the eigenvector for the first principal component: income = .497; education = .533; occupational prestige = .554; median home value = .403). Next, the investigators estimated a series of Cox proportional hazards models using one socioeconomic-status variable at a time in equations including age and sex on the right-hand side. To facilitate comparison of the strength of each variable in explaining mortality hazard, standardized scores on the variables were used (mean = 0; standard deviation = 1). All cancers examined in Chapter 7 (lung, prostate, and cervix) were combined in stratified Cox equations. Betas on these variables were as follows: income = $-.143$ (s.e. = .069); education = $-.154$ (s.e. = .060); occupational prestige = $-.067$ (s.e. = .059); median home value = $-.008$ (s.e. = .059). Clearly, income and education were the best predictors. Multi-item socioeconomic-status indicators comprising sums of standardized scores on (1) income and education; (2) income, education, and occupational prestige; and (3) income, education, occupational prestige, and median home value were entered into Cox equations. The income-education combination produced the highest betas and lowest p values. Clearly, a focus on income and education appeared to support the most efficient analysis.

The analysis summarized in Chapter 7 utilized both a simple scale combining income and education, and income and education as separate independent variables. The multi-item scale was used to provide an overview of the relation between socioeconomic status and mortality. Most of the analysis used equations with income and education entered as separate variables, to determine whether they had differing effects. In the tables that follow, income and education were entered into the same equations, so that results would reflect the effect of income after education had explained all it could, and vice versa. Income and education were moderately related (Pearson's $r = .358$).

Equations in this phase of the analysis add a contextual variable to the right-hand side of the equations beyond those of Chapters 5 and 6: urban versus rural location. Availability of adequate health services in rural areas was a major concern of researchers in the 1970s and 1980s. The contributions of income and education to survival or to postulated intervening variables constituting health services (for instance, detection at a routine physical or intensive therapy) could not be assessed adequately without controlling for the urban or rural nature of the subject's residence.

Table B-7.1 provides an overview of the relation between socioeconomic status and mortality in lung, prostate, and cervical cancer. The table presents logistic regression equations predicting five-year survival. Socioeconomic status is represented as a multi-item indicator based on the sum of standardized scores on income and education. This index is entered as three dummy variables representing the highest three quartiles; each dummy variable represents the difference in mortality risk from the lowest quartile, omitted from the equation. Percentage changes in mortality risk reflected in Figure 7 in the text are computed on the basis of the coefficients in Table B-7.1.

The rest of the analysis summarized in Chapter 7 includes income and education in equations of various kinds as separate, continuous variables. Tables B-7.2 and B-7.3 model what may be considered "intervening variables" linking socioeconomic status and survival versus mortality through the processes of detection and treatment. Table B-7.2 presents coefficients from ordinary least squares equations predicting stage at diagnosis and number of treatment modalities, both continuous variables.

Table B-7.1 *Socioeconomic Status and Five-Year Survival:*
Logistic Regression (Standard Errors in Parentheses)

	All Sites	Lung	Prostate	Cervix
Socioeconomic Status				
II	.313	.197	.375	.743
	(.283)	(.407)	(.421)	(.965)
III	.210	−.455	.810	.844
	(.288)	(.480)	(.449)	(.831)
IV (highest)	.904**	.561	1.566**	.449
	(.298)	(.419)	(.490)	(1.099)
Patient Characteristic				
Sex	.743*	.690*	—	—
	(.312)	(.317)		
Age	−.018	−.031	.030	−.039
	(.012)	(.016)	(.025)	(.027)
Urban	.016	−.006	.281	−.901
	(.310)	(.482)	(.481)	(.842)
Cancer Site				
Prostate	2.320**	—	—	—
	(.286)			
Cervix	1.345**	—	—	—
	(.421)			

$*p < .05$
$**p < .01$

Table B-7.2 *Socioeconomic Status, Detection, and Treatment: Regression Coefficients (Standard Errors in Parentheses)*

	Dependent Variable	
	Stage at Detection	*Number of Treatment Modalities*
A. All Sites		
Socioeconomic Dimension		
Income	.001	.031**
	(.014)	(.010)
Education	−.029*	−.010
	(.013)	(.010)
Patient Characteristic		
Sex	−.244*	.003
	(.119)	(.086)
Age	.006	−.009**
	(.005)	(.003)
Urban	−.112	.029
	(.121)	(.088)
Cancer Stage	—	.137**
		(.036)
Cancer Site		
Prostate	−.437**	−.243**
	(.102)	(.075)
Cervix	−.447*	−.145
	(.174)	(.127)
$R^2 =$	.11	.15
B. Lung		
Socioeconomic Dimension		
Income	.004	.004
	(.021)	(.014)
Education	−.007	.000
	(.022)	(.015)
Patient Characteristic		
Sex	−.257*	−.033
	(.119)	(.082)
Age	.009	−.009*
	(.006)	(.004)
Urban	−.165	.094
	(.177)	(.121)

		Dependent Variable	
		Stage at Detection	*Number of Treatment Modalities*
Cancer Stage		—	.141**
			(.050)
	$R^2 =$	.04	.07
C. Prostate			
Socioeconomic Dimension			
Income		−.017	.044**
		(.023)	(.017)
Education		−.045*	−.020
		(.019)	(.014)
Patient Characteristic			
Age		−.008	−.009
		(.010)	(.007)
Urban		−.217	.007
		(.211)	(.154)
Cancer Stage		—	.106
			(.056)
	$R^2 =$	.05	.10
D. Cervix			
Socioeconomic Dimension			
Income		.021	.085*
		(.035)	(.033)
Education		−.010	.022
		(.031)	(.029)
Patient Characteristic			
Age		.016*	−.014*
		(.007)	(.007)
Urban		.265	−.084
		(.206)	(.196)
Cancer Stage		—	.456
			(.153)
	$R^2 =$	.15	.38

$*p < .05$
$**p < .01$

Table B-7.3 *Socioeconomic Status, Detection, and Treatment:*
Logistic Regression (Standard Errors in Parentheses)

	Dependent Variable	
	Detected at Routine Physical	*Received Surgery*
A. All Sites		
Socioeconomic Dimension		
Income	.096**	.043
	(.035)	(.039)
Education	.095**	−.079*
	(.035)	(.037)
Patient Characteristic		
Sex	.057	.595
	(.321)	(.330)
Age	.014	−.018
	(.012)	(.013)
Urban	−.146	−.570
	(.317)	(.355)
Cancer Stage	—	−.737**
		(.140)
Cancer Site		
Prostate	.555*	−.413
	(.280)	(.278)
Cervix	.561	−.116
	(.460)	(.539)
B. Lung		
Socioeconomic Dimension		
Income	.036	.002
	(.058)	(.071)
Education	.133*	−.016
	(.062)	(.070)
Patient Characteristic		
Sex	.508	.445
	(.330)	(.395)
Age	.028	.026
	(.018)	(.020)
Urban	.625	−.104
	(.580)	(.582)
Cancer Stage	—	−1.884**
		(.286)

	Dependent Variable	
	Detected at Routine Physical	*Received Surgery*
C. Prostate		
Socioeconomic Dimension		
Income	.149**	.041
	(.055)	(.055)
Education	.092	−.096*
	(.047)	(.048)
Patient Characteristic		
Age	.008	−.055*
	(.024)	(.025)
Urban	−.195	−.845
	(.517)	(.535)
Cancer Stage	—	−.077
		(.185)
D. Cervix		
Socioeconomic Dimension		
Income	−.025	.497
	(.137)	(.296)
Education	−.049	−.030
	(.129)	(.199)
Patient Characteristic		
Age	−.020	−.085
	(.029)	(.055)
Urban	−1.834*	−7.817
	(.828)	(21.292)
Cancer Stage	—	−.913
		(.962)

*p < .05
**p < .01

Table B-7.4 *Income, Education, and Relative Mortality Risk:*
Proportional Hazards Models

	B Coeff.	Risk Ratio	Std. Error	Confidence Limits		p Value
				Lower	*Upper*	
A. All Sites						
Income	−.040	.961	.025	.915	1.009	.11
Education	−.047	.954	.022	.914	.996	.03
Urban	−.181	.834	.188	.575	1.210	.33
Sex	−.448	.639	.161	.465	.879	<.01
Age	.010	1.010	.008	.995	1.026	.18
B. Lung						
Income	−.052	.949	.031	.893	1.009	.09
Education	.005	1.005	.030	.947	1.067	.85
Urban	−.039	.962	.245	.592	1.562	.87
Sex	−.458	.633	.163	.458	.874	<.01
Age	.010	1.010	.009	.993	1.028	.24
C. Prostate						
Income	−.041	.960	.046	.877	1.051	.37
Education	−.116	.891	.034	.832	.954	<.01
Urban	−.558	.573	.309	.310	1.056	.07
Age	−.008	.992	.020	.953	1.032	.68
D. Cervix						
Income	−.093	.911	.141	.689	1.205	.51
Education	−.077	.926	.105	.751	1.141	.47
Urban	.521	1.684	.892	.288	9.849	.56
Age	.039	1.040	.024	.991	1.091	.11

Table B-7.5 *Income, Education, and Relative Mortality Risk:*
Proportional Hazards Models, Including Stage

	B Coeff.	Risk Ratio	Std. Error	Confidence Limits Lower	Upper	p Value
A. All Sites						
Income	−.053	.948	.028	.898	1.002	.05
Education	−.039	.962	.024	.918	1.009	.10
Urban	−.133	.876	.206	.582	1.318	.52
Sex	−.504	.604	.178	.425	.860	<.01
Age	−.003	.997	.008	.981	1.014	.74
Cancer Stage	.799	2.224	.088	1.867	2.648	<.01
B. Lung						
Income	−.073	.929	.036	.865	.998	<.05
Education	.007	1.007	.034	.941	1.077	.85
Urban	−.067	.935	.276	.542	1.615	.81
Sex	−.534	.586	.183	.408	.842	<.01
Age	−.003	.997	.010	.978	1.016	.77
Cancer Stage	.689	1.992	.114	1.588	2.498	<.01
C. Prostate						
Income	−.039	.961	.048	.874	1.058	.42
Education	−.090	.914	.037	.849	.983	<.02
Urban	−.243	.784	.341	.399	1.540	.47
Age	−.020	.981	.020	.943	1.020	.32
Cancer Stage	.860	2.363	.144	1.776	3.144	<.01
D. Cervix						
Income	−.307	.735	.189	.506	1.070	.10
Education	−.074	.929	.102	.759	1.135	.47
Urban	−.681	.506	.929	.080	3.185	.47
Age	.005	1.005	.028	.951	1.062	.87
Cancer Stage	2.675	N.A.	.798	N.A.	N.A.	<.01

Table B-7.3, including the same right-hand variables, presents logistic regression coefficients from equations predicting detection at a routine physical and surgery as part of treatment received, both dichotomous variables.

Tables B-7.4 and B-7.5 focus on mortality risk itself. These tables present beta coefficients and other statistics from Cox equations. Table B-7.4 presents a model without stage; Table B-7.5 presents a model with stage included on the right-hand side.

Two additional sets of proportional hazards models were estimated for more detailed analyses of two cancers. The first set was run on lung cancer cases with histologies other than small or oat cell carcinoma, and omits Stage III cases and patients over sixty-five years of age whatever the histology. In a model estimated with sex, age, rural versus urban residence, income, and education on the right-hand side, income had a coefficient of $-.134$ (s.e. $= .062, p < .05$). When stage was added to the right-hand side, the coefficient for income became $-.148$ (s.e. $= .073$, $p < .05$).

The second set was run on all cases of prostate cancer accrued, but includes detection-related intervening variables to help explain the relation between education and mortality risk. In an equation including the right-hand variables of age, rural versus urban residence, income, education, detection at a routine physical, and pain at time of detection, the coefficient on education was $-.090$ (s.e. $= .034, p < .01$). When stage was added to the right-hand side, the coefficient on education became $-.086$ (s.e. $= .037, p < .02$).

Chapter 8: The Health Maintenance Organization

This chapter attempts to determine whether and in what manner membership in Group Health Cooperative of Puget Sound affected treatment and survival of patients with lung, prostate, and cervical cancer diagnosed in King and Pierce Counties, Washington, between 1980 and 1982.

In all analyses presented or summarized in Chapter 8, membership in Group Health Cooperative served as the independent variable. Statistical analyses were similar to those performed in the preceding chapters.

Multivariate models, whether ordinary least squares, logistic multiple regression, or Cox proportional hazards, included the following variables on the right-hand side: age, education, income, and urban versus rural location of residence. Stage is included in most models, except, of course, the models predicting stage itself.

All individuals identified as HMO members in this part of the SLACS belonged to Group Health Cooperative of Puget Sound. Between 1980 and 1982, Group Health Cooperative was the only HMO operating in northwest Washington State. About 15 percent of the subjects interviewed in the SLACS and the populations of King and Pierce Counties were Group Health Cooperative enrollees. Data published by the Puget Sound Health Systems Agency[7] and discussions with local health care providers indicate that only two other organizations, both independent practice associations (IPAs), offered services outside fee-for-service settings during the data collection period. The total enrollment of these organizations amounted to considerably less than 1 percent of the populations of King and Pierce Counties. Thus, the assumption that virtually all those not belonging to the Group Health Cooperative received fee-for-service care appears reasonable. Almost no HMO members reported paying for care out of pocket, suggesting that few, if any, sought outside care for their cancers.

Research findings summarized in Chapter 8 are based on Tables B-8.1 through B-8.6. Table B-8.1 presents coefficients from ordinary least squares equations predicting three delay-related variables. Statistically significant results were obtained on only one delay-related variable, time elapsed from diagnosis to first anticancer treatment. Group Health Cooperative membership predicts longer waiting time on this dimension for all cancer sites, with statistically significant coefficients also obtained for prostatic and cervical cancer.

Table B-8.2 presents coefficients from logistic regression equations predicting surgical treatment and multimodal treatment. HMO membership is not a statistically significant predictor of either of these dependent variables, presented as indices of "intensity of care" in Chapter 8.

Table B-8.3 presents coefficients from logistic equations predicting five-year survival as a dichotomous variable. This table forms the basis for the top panel in Figure 8. The table reports a positive relation between HMO membership and survival for prostate cancer (statistically significant), but a negative relation for lung and cervix (neither statistically significant). The coefficient on HMO membership in the equation based on all three cancers combined is not statistically significant.

Table B-8.1 *HMO Membership and Initiation of Care:*
Regression Coefficients (Standard Errors in Parentheses)

	Dependent Variable		
	Stage at Detection	*Time from Suspicion to Diagnosis*	*Time from Diagnosis to Treatment*
A. All Sites			
Patient Characteristic			
HMO Member	−.019	−.552	.563**
	(.130)	(.550)	(.157)
Sex	−.139	.130	−.134
	(.133)	(.562)	(.160)
Age	.004	−.011	.003
	(.005)	(.022)	(.006)
Education	−.002	−.126	.002
	(.016)	(.067)	(.019)
Income	.000	.078	.020
	(.017)	(.070)	(.020)
Urban	.021	.055	−.069
	(.150)	(.633)	(.180)
Cancer Stage	—	—	−.032
			(.071)
Cancer Site			
Prostate	−.452**	1.309**	.415**
	(.117)	(.495)	(.145)
Cervix	−.599**	.568	.544*
	(.193)	(.814)	(.236)
$R^2 =$	.11	.05	.13
B. Lung			
Patient Characteristic			
HMO Member	.112	−.455	.153
	(.193)	(.529)	(.150)
Sex	−.149	.074	−.130
	(.133)	(.356)	(.104)
Age	.007	−.012	.000
	(.007)	(.020)	(.006)
Education	.018	−.009	.019
	(.025)	(.068)	(.019)
Income	.006	.121	.032
	(.023)	(.064)	(.018)
Urban	−.168	−.299	.233
	(.216)	(.592)	(.168)

	Dependent Variable		
	Stage at Detection	*Time from Suspicion to Diagnosis*	*Time from Diagnosis to Treatment*
Cancer Stage	—	—	.050
			(.065)
$R^2 =$	.03	.05	.08

C. Prostate

Patient Characteristic

HMO Member	−.028	−.734	.543*
	(.211)	(1.124)	(.262)
Age	−.013	−.014	.015
	(.012)	(.066)	(.015)
Education	−.016	−.218	−.030
	(.026)	(.137)	(.032)
Income	−.024	−.008	.014
	(.029)	(.154)	(.036)
Urban	.061	.218	.160
	(.305)	(1.625)	(.379)
Cancer Stage	—	—	−.069
			(.125)
$R^2 =$	.02	.04	.07

D. Cervix

Patient Characteristic

HMO Member	−.316	1.062	3.138**
	(.370)	(1.910)	(.882)
Age	.014	.000	−.004
	(.008)	(.040)	(.019)
Education	−.007	−.103	.068
	(.034)	(.177)	(.081)
Income	.034	.147	−.068
	(.040)	(.207)	(.096)
Urban	.379	.680	−.936
	(.228)	(1.175)	(.561)
Cancer Stage	—	—	.111
			(.430)
$R^2 =$	.18	.05	.39

$*p < .05$
$**p < .01$

Table B-8.2 *HMO Membership and Cancer Treatment:*
Logistic Regression (Standard Errors in Parentheses)

	Dependent Variable	
	Surgery	Multimodal Treatment
A. All Sites		
Patient Characteristic		
HMO Member	−.399	−.123
	(.299)	(.327)
Sex	.586	.080
	(.331)	(.320)
Age	−.017	−.029*
	(.013)	(.013)
Education	−.075*	−.029
	(.037)	(.039)
Income	.043	.096*
	(.039)	(.040)
Urban	−.567	.242
	(.356)	(.348)
Cancer Stage	−.741**	.513**
	(.140)	(.143)
Cancer Site		
Prostate	−.386	−.553
	(.279)	(.291)
Cervix	−.114	−.342
	(.538)	(.484)
B. Lung		
Patient Characteristic		
HMO Member	−.536	−.888
	(.578)	(.555)
Sex	.429	−.076
	(.398)	(.334)
Age	.027	−.027
	(.020)	(.017)
Education	−.016	−.003
	(.069)	(.060)
Income	.004	.003
	(.071)	(.059)
Urban	−.056	.386
	(.583)	(.505)
Cancer Stage	−1.897**	.627**
	(.287)	(.208)

	Dependent Variable	
	Surgery	Multimodal Treatment
C. Prostate		
Patient Characteristic		
HMO Member	−.537	.283
	(.387)	(.442)
Age	−.054*	−.025
	(.026)	(.028)
Education	−.089	−.072
	(.048)	(.058)
Income	.039	.143*
	(.055)	(.063)
Urban	−.089	.395
	(.543)	(.627)
Cancer Stage	−.072	.299
	(.186)	(.218)
D. Cervix		
Patient Characteristic		
HMO Member	6.063	.868
	N.A.	(1.460)
Age	−.083	−.096
	(.054)	(.053)
Education	−.028	.047
	(.198)	(.185)
Income	.477	.447*
	(.299)	(.189)
Urban	−8.833	−.491
	(21.375)	(1.078)
Cancer Stage	−.871	2.128*
	(.963)	(.920)

$*p < .05$
$**p < .01$

Table B-8.3 *HMO Membership and Five-Year Survival, Direct Effects Only:*
Logistic Regression (Standard Errors in Parentheses)

	All Sites	Lung	Prostate	Cervix
Patient Characteristic				
HMO Member	.357	−.519	1.010*	−1.707
	(.352)	(.656)	(.494)	(1.500)
Sex	.650	.701	—	—
	(.374)	(.390)		
Age	−.015	−.019	.017	−.037
	(.014)	(.020)	(.029)	(.033)
Education	.055	−.026	.112	.026
	(.043)	(.074)	(.059)	(.141)
Income	.068	.120	.077	.101
	(.044)	(.068)	(.068)	(.190)
Urban	−.184	−.288	−.172	.427
	(.374)	(.551)	(.619)	(.930)
Cancer Stage	−1.173**	−1.139**	−1.172**	−1.927*
	(.157)	(.258)	(.215)	(.806)
Cancer Site				
Prostate	2.001**	—	—	—
	(.336)			
Cervix	.765	—	—	—
	(.512)			

*p < .05
**p < .01

Table B-8.4 *HMO Membership and Relative Mortality Risk: Proportional Hazards Models*

	Coeff.	Risk Ratio	Std. Error	Confidence Limits		p Value
				Lower	Upper	
A. All Sites						
HMO Member	−.385	.681	.213	.447	1.038	.07
Sex	−.532	.588	.179	.412	.837	<.01
Age	−.003	.997	.008	.981	1.014	.75
Education	−.037	.963	.024	.919	1.010	.12
Income	−.057	.944	.028	.894	.997	.03
Urban	−.140	.870	.207	.577	1.310	.50
Cancer Stage	.809	2.245	.088	1.884	2.675	<.01
B. Lung						
HMO Member	.026	1.027	.268	.604	1.744	.92
Sex	−.532	.587	.184	.408	.845	<.01
Age	−.003	.997	.010	.978	1.016	.77
Education	.006	1.006	.034	.941	1.077	.84
Income	−.073	.929	.036	.865	.998	.04
Urban	−.068	.934	.276	.540	1.614	.80
Cancer Stage	.689	1.992	.114	1.588	2.498	<.01
C. Prostate						
HMO Member	−.973	.378	.351	.189	.757	<.01
Age	−.016	.984	.020	.946	1.023	.41
Education	−.086	.918	.038	.852	.989	.02
Income	−.054	.948	.048	.862	1.042	.26
Urban	−.345	.708	.347	.356	1.408	.31
Cancer Stage	.906	2.473	.145	1.858	3.293	<.01
D. Cervix						
HMO Member	4.090	59.734	1.760	1.833	1946.772	.02
Age	.009	1.009	.028	.955	1.066	.74
Education	−.109	.897	.102	.733	1.097	.28
Income	−.450	.638	.208	.423	.963	.03
Urban	−1.306	.271	1.081	.032	2.302	.22
Cancer Stage	3.497	33.009	1.019	4.391	248.118	<.01

Table B-8.5 *HMO Membership and Five-Year Survival, HMO-Income Interactions: Logistic Regression (Standard Errors in Parentheses)*

	All Sites	Lung	Prostate	Cervix
Patient Characteristic				
Sex	.569	.598	—	—
	(.356)	(.376)		
Age	−.016	−.010	.005	−.039
	(.013)	(.019)	(.030)	(.032)
Education	.058	−.032	.119*	.051
	(.040)	(.069)	(.058)	(.138)
Urban	−.143	−.132	−.055	−.312
	(.362)	(.553)	(.609)	(.916)
Income				
Middle	.402	.513	.539	−.001
	(.308)	(.427)	(.513)	(.951)
High	.613	.703	.813	1.798
	(.374)	(.572)	(.587)	(1.929)
HMO Member				
Low Income	1.319*	.096	1.987*	3.976
	(.528)	(.946)	(.766)	(25.014)
Mid Income	−.144	−.911	.330	N.A.
	(.654)	(1.199)	(.944)	
High Income	−.779	−.989	−.288	−3.752
	(.643)	(1.306)	(.881)	(2.484)
Cancer Stage	−1.231**	−1.233**	−1.147**	−2.044*
	(.157)	(.258)	(.216)	(.814)
Cancer Site				
Prostate	1.971**	—	—	—
	(.323)			
Cervix	.753	—	—	—
	(.475)			

*$p < .05$
**$p < .01$

Table B-8.6 *HMO Membership–Income-Level Interactions: Proportional Hazards Models*

	Coeff.	Risk Ratio	Std. Error	Confidence Limits		p Value
				Lower	*Upper*	
A. All Sites						
Sex	−.528	.590	.173	.419	.830	<.01
Age	−.002	.998	.008	.982	1.014	.78
Education	−.041	.960	.023	.918	1.004	.07
Urban	−.176	.839	.204	.560	1.255	.38
Income						
Middle	−.398	.672	.170	.480	.940	<.01
High	−.331	.718	.223	.462	1.117	.13
HMO Member						
Low Income	−.844	.430	.312	.232	.798	<.01
Mid Income	.190	1.209	.361	.592	2.470	.59
High Income	.145	1.156	.451	.473	2.825	.74
Cancer Stage	.844	2.327	.087	1.960	2.762	<.01
B. Lung						
Sex	−.515	.597	.177	.421	.848	<.01
Age	−.005	.995	.009	.977	1.013	.57
Education	.002	1.002	.031	.942	1.066	.94
Urban	−.115	.891	.272	.521	1.526	.67
Income						
Middle	−.371	.690	.203	.461	1.032	.06
High	−.319	.727	.290	.409	1.290	.27
HMO Member						
Low Income	−.162	.850	.376	.404	1.791	.66
Mid Income	.320	1.377	.437	.580	3.271	.46
High Income	.032	1.033	.761	.229	4.661	.96
Cancer Stage	.721	2.057	.112	1.647	2.569	<.01
C. Prostate						
Age	−.010	.990	.021	.949	1.032	.63
Education	−.093	.912	.037	.847	.982	.02
Urban	−.450	.638	.352	.318	1.281	.20
Income						
Middle	−.411	.663	.336	.341	1.289	.22
High	−.575	.563	.414	.248	1.278	.16
HMO Member						
Low Income	−1.702	.182	.541	.062	.533	<.01
Mid Income	−.135	.873	.652	.240	3.174	.83
High Income	.044	1.045	.651	.288	3.792	.94
Cancer Stage	.915	2.496	.143	1.881	3.313	<.01

Continued on next page

Table B-8.6 *Continued*

	Coeff.	Risk Ratio	Std. Error	Confidence Limits Lower	Upper	p Value
D. Cervix						
Age	.012	1.012	.027	.960	1.067	.65
Education	.060	1.061	.081	.904	1.247	.46
Urban	−.232	.793	.914	.130	4.844	.79
Income						
Middle	−.738	.478	.929	.076	3.010	.42
High	−1.051	.350	1.153	.036	3.429	.36
HMO Member						
Low Income	−6.141	.002	69.9065	N.A.	N.A.	.93
Mid Income			(None observed)			
High Income	2.671	14.461	1.626	.579	361.502	.10
Cancer Stage	2.103	8.194	.638	2.317	28.982	<.01

Table B-8.4 addresses the same issue as Table B-8.3, except that coefficients (from Cox proportional hazards models) reflect relative risk over the follow-up period for each patient. Statistically significant results in this table indicate that prostate cancer patients in the HMO have a lower risk of mortality over the course of the study than those in fee-for-service; cervical cancer patients in the HMO, however, have a higher risk (a finding based on only three HMO members). Mortality risk among lung cancer patients and all patients combined does not evidence a statistically significant association with HMO membership.

Equations summarized in Tables B-8.5 and B-8.6 include a series of interaction terms: HMO member vs. fee-for-service, low income; HMO member vs. fee-for-service, middle income; HMO member vs. fee-for-service, high income. Low income was under $20,000 per family in the year preceding the interview; middle income was $20,000–$34,999; high income was $35,000 and above. Coefficients on these variables represent the difference between HMO members and fee-for-service patients within each income category with respect to five-year survival (Table B-8.5) or relative mortality risk (Table B-8.6).

Table B-8.5 provides the basis for the bottom panel of Figure 8, presenting coefficients from logistic regression equations predicting five-year survival. For all the cancers analyzed, the coefficient on HMO membership *in the low-income category* is positive and statistically significant, indicating a greater likelihood of five-year survival for low-income HMO members. In equations based on individual cancers, this coefficient is statistically significant only for prostatic cancer. In cervical cancer, the standard error on the estimated coefficient is quite large; thus, the difference in five-year survival suggested is not definitive. However, the sign is positive in all disease-specific equations, supporting a generalization that, among the cancers studied here, low-income people have a better survival chance in an HMO than in fee-for-service. Nearly the same results are found in Table B-8.6, which presents Cox proportional hazards model coefficients.

Additional Cox proportional hazards models similar to those reported in Table B-8.6 were run, based on all cancers. One equation was based only on HMO members and fee-for-service patients who reported making out-of-pocket payments. The HMO member–low-income interaction term had a coefficient of $-.714$ (s.e. $= .330$). In the second equation, based on only HMO members and fee-for-service patients who made *no* payments, the coefficient was $-.978$ (s.e. $= .339$). These findings argue against two explanations for the observed benefits of HMO membership: (1) that payment accounts for the difference (as opposed to some characteristic of the HMO as a delivery system) or (2) that the "free" fee-for-service patients are destitute people, for whom any readily available source of care (fee-for-service *or* HMO) would improve chances for survival.

Notes

Preface

1. H. P. Greenwald, M. Bergner, and J. J. Bonica, "The Prevalence of Pain in Four Cancers," *Cancer* 60 (1987): 201–7.

2. H. P. Greenwald et al., "Work Disability among Cancer Patients," *Social Science and Medicine* 29 (1989): 1253–59.

Chapter 1

1. S. M. Shortell, "Factors Associated with the Use of Health Services," in *Introduction to Health Services,* ed. S. J. Williams and P. R. Torrens (New York: Wiley, 1984).

2. American Cancer Society, *Cancer Facts and Figures, 1986* (New York: American Cancer Society, 1986).

3. *Wall Street Journal,* November 12, 1986, p. 37.

4. B. N. Ames, R. Magaw, and L. S. Gold, "Ranking Possible Carcinogenic Hazards," *Science* 236 (1987): 271–80.

5. N. Cousins, *Anatomy of an Illness as Perceived by the Patient* (New York: Norton, 1979).

6. J. W. Worden and H. J. Sobel, "Ego Strength and Psychosocial Adaptation to Cancer," *Psychosomatic Medicine* 40 (1978): 485–592.

7. P. Maguire, "The Will to Live in the Cancer Patient," in *Mind and Cancer Prognosis,* ed. B. A. Stoll (New York: Wiley, 1978).

8. O. C. Simonton, S. Matthews-Simonton, and T. F. Sparks, "Psychological Interventions in the Treatment of Cancer," *Psychosomatics* 21 (1980): 226–33.

9. Cousins, *Anatomy of an Illness.*

10. H. P. Greenwald, *Social Problems in Cancer Control* (Cambridge, Mass.: Ballinger, 1980).

11. P. R. Torrens, "Historical Evolution and Overview of Health Services in the United States," in *Introduction to Health Services,* p. 5.

12. Ibid.

13. Ibid.

14. M. Stern, "The Recent Decline in Ischemic Heart Disease Mortality," *Annals of Internal Medicine* 91 (1979): 630–40.

15. American Cancer Society, *Cancer Facts and Figures.*

16. Ibid.

17. Ibid.

18. Ibid.

19. R. H. Brook et al., "Does Free Care Improve Adults' Health? Results from a Randomized Controlled Trial," *New England Journal of Medicine* 309 (1983): 1426–34.

20. A. L. Siu et al., "Inappropriate Use of Hospitals in a Randomized Trial of Health Insurance Plans," *New England Journal of Medicine* 315 (1986): 1259–66.

21. L. D. Brown, *Politics and Health Care Organization: HMOs as Federal Policy* (Washington, D.C.: Brookings Institution, 1983).

22. W. G. Manning et al., "A Controlled Trial of the Effect of a Prepaid Group Practice on Use of Services," *New England Journal of Medicine* 310 (1984): 1505–10.

23. L. F. Rossiter and G. R. Wilensky, *Out of Pocket Expenditures for Ambulatory Care Services,* USDHHS Pub. no. (PHS) 82-3332 (Washington, D.C.: U.S. Government Printing Office, 1982).

24. P. J. Farley, *Private Health Insurance in the United States,* USDHHS Pub. no. (PHS) 86-3406 (Washington, D.C.: U.S. Government Printing Office, 1986).

25. G. L. Cafferata, *Private Health Insurance of the Medicare Population,* USDHHS Pub. no. (PHS) 84-3364 (Washington, D.C.: U.S. Government Printing Office, 1984).

26. A. McMillan, J. Lubitz, and M. Newton, "Trends in Physician Assignment Rates for Medicare Services, 1968–1985," *Health Care Financing Review* 7 (1985): 59–75.

27. J. D. Kasper, "Health Status and Utilization Differences by Medicaid Coverage and Income," *Health Care Financing Review* 7 (1986): 1–17.

28. H. E. Freeman et al., "Americans Report on Their Access to Health Care," *Health Affairs* 6 (1987): 6–18, at 14.

29. S. M. Shortell, "Factors Associated with the Use of Health Services," p. 66.

30. J. Howard, "Avoidable Mortality from Cervical Cancer: Exploring the Concept," *Social Science and Medicine* 24 (1987): 507–14.

31. B. S. Ward, "X Ray Screening for Breast Cancer Gains but High Fees Hamper Widespread Use," *Wall Street Journal,* July 30, 1985, sec. 2, p. 1.

Chapter 2

1. E. Farber, "Cancer Development and Its Natural History: A Cancer Prevention Perspective," *Cancer* 52 (1988): 1676–79.

2. American Cancer Society, *Cancer Facts and Figures—1990* (Atlanta: American Cancer Society, 1990).

3. Farber, "Cancer Development."

4. N. Martini and E. J. Beattie, "Results of Surgical Treatment in Stage I Lung Cancer," *Journal of Cardiovascular Surgery* 74 (1977): 499–505.

5. American Cancer Society, *Cancer Facts and Figures.*

6. J. L. Young et al., *Cancer Incidence and Mortality in the United States, 1973–1977,* NCI Monograph no. 57 (Bethesda, Md.: National Cancer Institute, 1981).

7. Z. Petrovice and R. A. Figlin, "Lung Cancer," in *Cancer Treatment,* 2nd ed., ed. C. M. Haskell (Philadelphia: Saunders, 1985), pp. 180–211.

8. U.S. General Accounting Office, *Cancer Patient Survival: What Progress Has Been Made?* (Washington, D.C.: U.S. General Accounting Office, 1987).

9. J. Cairns, "The Treatment of Diseases and the War against Cancer," *Scientific American* 253 (1985): 51–59.

10. C. F. Mountain, "Assessment of the Role of Surgery for Control of Lung Cancer," *Annals of Thoracic Surgery* 24 (1977): 365–73.

11. Cairns, "The Treatment of Diseases."

12. H. P. Greenwald, "The Specificity of Quality-of-Life Measures among the Seriously Ill," *Medical Care* 25 (1987): 642–51.

13. "It's Over, Debbie," *Journal of the American Medical Association* 259 (1988): 272.

Chapter 3

1. J. Gunther, *Death Be Not Proud* (New York: Harper, 1949).

2. See, for example, C. M. Haskell, ed., *Cancer Treatment,* 2nd ed. (Philadelphia: Saunders, 1985); and V. T. DeVita, S. Hellman, and S. A. Rosenberg, *Principles and Practice of Oncology* (New York: Lippincott, 1982).

3. C. M. Haskell et al., "Breast Cancer," in *Cancer Treatment,* pp. 137–80.

4. P. H. Sugarbaker and S. Corlew, "Influence of Surgical Techniques on

Survival of Patients with Colorectal Cancer," *Diseases of the Colon and Rectum* 25 (1982): 545–57.

5. H. J. G. Bloom, "Radiotherapy," *Recent Results in Cancer Research* 78 (1981): 132–53.

6. J. T. Patterson, *The Dread Disease: Cancer and Modern American Culture* (Cambridge, Mass.: Harvard University Press, 1987).

7. G. Morstyn et al., "Small Cell Lung Cancer, 1973–1983: Early Progress and Recent Obstacles," *International Journal of Radiation: Oncology, Biology, Physics* 10 (1984): 515–39.

8. C. M. Haskell, "Principles of Cancer Chemotherapy," in *Cancer Treatment*, pp. 21–42.

9. Haskell et al., "Breast Cancer."

10. B. Cook and F. R. Watson, "A Comparison by Age of Death Due to Prostate Cancer Alone," *Journal of Urology* 100 (1968): 669–71.

11. J. H. Conant et al., "Radical Prostatectomy versus Radiation Therapy," *Urology* 25 (1985): 347–49.

12. D. F. Paulson et al., "Radical Surgery versus Radiotherapy for Adenocarcinoma of the Prostate," *Journal of Urology* 128 (1982): 502–4.

13. E. S. Levine et al., "Role of Transurethral Resection in Dissemination of Cancer of the Prostate," *Urology* 28 (1986): 179–83.

14. D. P. Byar, "The Veterans Administration Cooperative Urological Research Group's Studies of Cancer of the Prostate," *Cancer* 32 (1973): 1126–50.

15. C. F. Mountain, "Assessment of the Role of Surgery for Control of Lung Cancer," *Annals of Thoracic Surgery* 24 (1977): 365–73.

16. A. S. Lichter et al., "The Role of Radiation Therapy in the Treatment of Small Cell Lung Cancer," *Cancer* 55 (1985): 2163–75.

17. R. J. Ginsberg et al., "Modern Thirty-Day Operative Mortality for Surgical Resections in Lung Cancer," *Journal of Thoracic and Cardiovascular Surgery* 86 (1983): 654–58.

18. Lichter, "The Role of Radiation Therapy."

19. R. J. Weiss and W. E. Lucas, "Adenocarcinoma of the Uterine Cervix," *Cancer* 57 (1985): 1996–2001.

20. R. A. Malt, "Treatment of Pancreatic Cancer," *Journal of the American Medical Association* 250 (1983): 1433–37.

21. M. Chase, "To Doctor and Patient, Test of a New Drug Is a Turbulent Experience," *Wall Street Journal*, September 26, 1985.

22. Haskell, "Principles of Cancer Chemotherapy."

23. U.S. Department of Health and Human Services, *Understanding the Immune System*, USDHHS Pub. no. (NIH) 88-529 (Washington, D.C.: U.S. Government Printing Office, 1988).

24. A. D. Kaluzny et al., "Evaluating Organizational Design to Assure Technology Transfer: The Case of the Community Clinical Oncology Program," *Journal of the National Cancer Institute* 81 (1989): 1717–25.

25. R. L. Stephens et al., "Adriamycin and Cyclophosphamide versus Hydroxyurea in Advanced Prostate Cancer," *Cancer* 53 (1984): 406–10.

26. M. Pavone-Macaluso, G. deVoogt, and G. Viggiano, "Comparison of

DES, Cyprosterone Acetate, and Medroxyprogesterone Acetate in Advanced Prostate Cancer," *Journal of Urology* 136 (1986): 624–31.

27. J. C. Ruckdeschel et al., "Chemotherapy for Metastatic Non–Small Cell Bronchogenic Carcinoma: Cyclophosphamide, Doxorubicin, and Etoposide versus Mitomycin and Vinblastine (EST 2575, Generation IV)," *Cancer Treatment Reports* 68 (1984): 1325–29; J. C. Ruckdeschel et al., "A Randomized Trial of the Four Most Active Regimens for Metastatic Non–Small Cell Lung Cancer," *Journal of Clinical Oncology* 4 (1986): 14–22; D. M. Finkelstein, D. S. Ettinger, and J. C. Ruckdeschel, "Long Term Survivors in Metastatic Non–Small Cell Lung Cancer: An ECOG Study," *Journal of Clinical Oncology* 4 (1986): 702–9.

28. Ruckdeschel et al., "A Randomized Trial," p. 22.

29. Morstyn, "Small Cell Lung Cancer."

30. M. C. Perry et al., "Chemotherapy with or without Radiation Therapy in Limited Small Cell Carcinoma of the Lung," *New England Journal of Medicine* 316 (1987): 912–18.

31. S. A. Rosenberg et al., "A Progress Report on the Treatment of 157 Patients with Advanced Cancer Using Lymphokine-Activated Killer Cells and Interleukin-2 or High Dose Interleukin-2 Alone," *New England Journal of Medicine* 316 (1987): 889–97.

32. M. Chase, "FDA Advises Delay in Recommendation on Cetus Drug against Kidney Cancer," *Wall Street Journal,* July 31, 1990.

33. B. R. Cassileth, "Social Implications of Alternative Cancer Therapies," in *Proceedings of the Fifth National Conference on Human Values and Cancer* (New York: American Cancer Society, 1987), pp. 63–66.

34. C. G. Moertel, "A Trial of Laetrile Now," *New England Journal of Medicine* 298 (1978): 218.

35. C. G. Moertel et al., "A Clinical Trial of Amygdalin (Laetrile) in the Treatment of Human Cancer," *New England Journal of Medicine* 306 (1982): 201–6.

36. Ibid.

37. E. T. Creagan et al., "Failure of High-Dose Vitamin C (Ascorbic Acid) Therapy to Benefit Patients with Advanced Cancer," *New England Journal of Medicine* 301 (1979): 687–90.

38. C. G. Moertel et al., "High Dose Vitamin C versus Placebo in the Treatment of Patients with Advanced Cancer Who Had No Prior Chemotherapy," *New England Journal of Medicine* 312 (1985): 137–41.

39. L. Pauling and C. G. Moertel, "A Proposition: Megadoses of Vitamin C Are Valuable in the Treatment of Cancer" (Debate), *Nutrition Review* 44 (1986): 28–32.

40. B. R. Cassileth et al., "Contemporary Unorthodox Treatments in Cancer Medicine," *Annals of Internal Medicine* 101 (1984): 105–12.

41. R. K. Oldham, "Patient-Funded Cancer Research," *New England Journal of Medicine* 316 (1987): 46–47.

42. W. J. Broad, "Fraud in Science Taints the High and Mighty," *New York Times,* March 20, 1983.

43. P. Weiss, "Conduct Unbecoming," *New York Times,* October 29, 1989.

44. P. J. Hilts, "Crucial Data Were Fabricated in Report Signed by Top Biologist," *New York Times,* March 21, 1991.

45. J. Maddox, "Dr. Baltimore's Experiment in Hubris," *New York Times,* March 31, 1991.

46. W. J. Mackillop, G. K. Ward, and B. O'Sullivan, "The Use of Expert Surrogates to Evaluate Clinical Trials in Non–Small Cell Lung Cancer," *British Journal of Cancer* 54 (1986): 661–67.

Chapter 4

1. E. Boyland, "The Correlation of Experimental Carcinogenesis and Cancer in Man," *Progress in Experimental Tumor Research* 11 (1967): 222–34.

2. R. Doll and R. Peto, "The Causes of Cancer: Quantitative Estimates of Avoidable Risks of Cancer in the United States Today," *Journal of the National Cancer Institute* 66 (1981): 1196–1308.

3. P. Decoufle, "Occupation," in *Cancer Epidemiology and Prevention,* ed. D. Schottenfeld and J. F. Fraumeni (Philadelphia: Saunders, 1982), pp. 318–35.

4. B. I. Weinstein, "The Scientific Basis for Carcinogen Detection and Primary Prevention of Cancer," *Cancer* 47 (1988): 1133–41.

5. Doll and Peto, "The Causes of Cancer."

6. B. N. Ames, R. Magaw, and L. S. Gold, "Ranking Possible Carcinogenic Hazards," *Science* 236 (1987): 271–80.

7. J. D. Boice and C. E. Land, "Ionizing Radiation," in *Cancer Epidemiology and Prevention,* pp. 231–53.

8. J. Scotto, T. R. Fears, and J. F. Fraumeni, "Solar Radiation," in *Cancer Epidemiology and Prevention,* pp. 254–76.

9. H. J. Geiger, "Generations of Poison and Lies," *New York Times,* August 5, 1990.

10. American Cancer Society, *Cancer Rates and Risks, 1990* (Atlanta: American Cancer Society, 1990).

11. Scotto, Fears, and Fraumeni, "Solar Radiation."

12. R. E. Rowland, A. F. Stehney, and H. F. Lucas, "Dose-Response Relationships for Female Radium Dial Workers," *Radiation Research* 76 (1978): 368–83.

13. V. E. Archer, J. D. Gillam, and J. K. Wagoner, "Respiratory Disease Mortality among Uranium Miners," *Annals of the New York Academy of Sciences* 271 (1976): 280–93.

14. Boice and Land, "Ionizing Radiation."

15. R. E. Shore, "Electromagnetic Radiation and Cancer: Cause and Prevention," *Cancer* 62 (1988): 1747–54.

16. Y. Shimizu, W. J. Schull, and H. Kato, "Cancer Risks among Atomic

Bomb Survivors," *Journal of the American Medical Association* 264 (1990): 601–4.

17. R. A. Conrad, "Summary of Thyroid Findings in Marshallese 22 Years after Exposure to Radioactive Fallout," in *Radiation-Associated Thyroid Carcinoma*, ed. L. De Groot (New York: Grune and Stratton, 1977), pp. 241–57.

18. G. G. Caldwell, D. B. Kelly, and C. W. Heath, "Leukemia among Participants in Military Maneuvers at a Nuclear Bomb Test: A Preliminary Report," *Journal of the American Medical Association* 244 (1980): 1575–78.

19. W. Stevens et al., "Leukemia in Utah and Radioactive Fallout from the Nevada Test Site," *Journal of the American Medical Association* 264 (1990): 285–91.

20. Shore, "Electromagnetic Radiation and Cancer."

21. National Council on Radiation Protection, *Evaluation of Occupational and Environmental Exposures to Radon and Radon Daughters in the United States* (Bethesda, Md.: National Council on Radiation Protection and Measurements, 1984).

22. Shore, "Electromagnetic Radiation and Cancer," p. 1748.

23. C. Robinette, C. Silverman, and S. Jablon, "Effects upon Health of Occupational Exposure to Microwave Radiation (Radar)," *American Journal of Epidemiology* 112 (1980): 39–53.

24. Doll and Peto, "The Causes of Cancer."

25. P. N. MacGee, R. Montesano, and R. Preussmann, "N-Nitroso Compounds and Related Carcinogens," in *Chemical Carcinogens*, ed. C. E. Searle (Washington, D.C.: American Chemical Society, 1976), pp. 491–625.

26. S. A. Yuspa and C. C. Harris, "Molecular and Cellular Basis of Chemical Carcinogenesis," in *Cancer Epidemiology and Prevention*, pp. 23–43.

27. P. C. MacDonald et al., "Effect of Obesity on Conversion of Plasma Androstenedione to Estrone in Premenopausal Women with and without Endometrial Cancer," *American Journal of Obstetrics and Gynecology* 130 (1978): 448–55.

28. B. E. Henderson, R. K. Ross, and L. Bernstein, "Estrogen as a Cause of Human Cancer: The Richard and Hilda Rosenthal Foundation Award Lecture," *Cancer Research* 48 (1988): 246–63.

29. E. A. Lew and L. Garfinkle, "Variations in Mortality by Weight among 750,000 Men and Women," *Journal of Chronic Diseases* 32 (1979): 563–76.

30. C. W. Welch, "Interrelationship between Dietary Fat and Endocrine Processes in Mammary Gland Tumorigenesis," *Progress in Clinical and Biological Research* 222 (1986): 623–54.

31. D. G. Zaridze, "Environmental Etiology of Large Bowel Cancer," *Journal of the National Cancer Institute* 70 (1983): 389–400.

32. T. Byers, "Diet and Cancer," *Cancer* 62 (1988): 1713–24.

33. J. Waterhouse et al., eds., *Cancer Incidence in Five Continents*, vol. 3 (Lyon: International Agency for Research on Cancer, 1976).

34. National Research Council, *Diet and Health* (Washington, D.C.: National Academy Press, 1989), p. 313.

35. Byers, "Diet and Cancer."

36. W. C. Willett et al., "Relation of Serum Vitamins A and E and Ca-

rotenoids to the Risk of Cancer," *New England Journal of Medicine* 310 (1984): 430–34; A. Paganini-Hill et al., "Vitamin A, Beta-Carotene, and Risk of Cancer: A Prospective Study," *Journal of the National Cancer Institute* 79 (1987): 443–48.

37. H. Trowell et al., "Dietary Fiber Redefined," *Lancet* 1 (1976): 967.

38. International Agency for Research on Cancer, Intestinal Microecology Group, "Dietary Fiber, Transit Time, Fecal Bacteria, Steroids, and Colon Cancer in Two Scandinavian Populations," *Lancet* 2 (1977): 207–11.

39. Byers, "Diet and Cancer."

40. National Research Council, *Diet and Health*, p. 299.

41. Ames, Magaw, and Gold, "Ranking Possible Carcinogenic Hazards."

42. Ibid.

43. National Research Council, *Diet and Health*, p. 594.

44. B. S. MacMahon et al., "Coffee and Cancer of the Pancreas," *New England Journal of Medicine* 304 (1981): 630–33.

45. C. C. Hsieh, B. S. MacMahon, and D. Yen, "Coffee and Cancer of the Pancreas (Chapter 2)," *New England Journal of Medicine* 315 (1986): 587–89.

46. R. K. Ross, A. Paganini-Hill, and B. E. Henderson, "Epidemiology of Prostate Cancer," in *Urological Cancer,* ed. D. G. Skinner (New York: Grune and Stratton, 1983).

47. Doll and Peto, "The Causes of Cancer," p. 1237.

48. R. K. Ross et al., "Avoidable Nondietary Risk Factors for Cancer," *American Family Practitioner* 38 (1988): 153–60.

49. L. Bernstein et al., "The Effects of Moderate Physical Activity on Menstrual Cycle Patterns in Adolescence: Implications for Breast Cancer Prevention," *British Journal of Cancer* 55 (1987): 681–85.

50. Byers, "Diet and Cancer."

51. Ross, "Avoidable Nondietary Risk Factors."

52. Doll and Peto, "The Causes of Cancer."

53. J. W. Horm et al., eds., *SEER Program: Cancer Incidence and Mortality in the United States, 1973–81,* USDHHS Pub. no. (NIH) 85-1837 (Washington, D.C.: U.S. Government Printing Office, 1984).

54. B. E. Henderson et al., "Endogenous Hormones as a Major Factor in Human Cancer," *Cancer Research* 42 (1982): 3232–39.

55. B. E. Henderson et al., "Elevated Serum Levels of Estrogen and Prolactin in Daughters of Patients with Breast Cancer," *New England Journal of Medicine* 293 (1975): 790–95.

56. R. Ghanadian, K. M. Puah, and E. P. M. O'Donoghue, "Serum Testosterone and Dihydrotestosterone in Carcinoma of the Prostate," *British Journal of Cancer* 39 (1979): 696–99.

57. K. P. Ramming and C. M. Haskell, "Colorectal Malignancies," in *Cancer Treatment,* 2nd ed., ed. C. M. Haskell (Philadelphia: Saunders, 1985), pp. 275–307.

58. G. R. Newell and V. G. Vogel, "Personal Risk Factors: What Do They Mean?" *Cancer* 62 (1988): 1695–1701.

59. M. Mori et al., "Reproductive, Genetic, and Dietary Risk Factors for Ovarian Cancer," *American Journal of Epidemiology* 128 (1988): 771–77.

60. W. K. Cavenee et al., "Prediction of Familial Predisposition to Retinoblastoma," *New England Journal of Medicine* 314 (1986): 1201–7.

61. N. E. Caporaso et al., "Lung Cancer and the Debrisoquine Metabolic Phenotype," and T. A. Sellers et al., "Evidence for Mendelian Inheritance in the Pathogenesis of Lung Cancer," *Journal of the National Cancer Institute* 82 (1990): 1264–72, 1272–79.

62. J. E. Bishop, "Gene That Spurs Lung Cancer Found," *Wall Street Journal*, August 15, 1990.

63. U.S. Department of Health and Human Services, *Cancer among Blacks and Other Minorities: Statistical Profiles*, USDHHS Pub. no. (NIH) 86-2785 (Washington, D.C.: U.S. Government Printing Office, 1986).

64. S. S. Devesa and E. L. Diamond, "Association of Breast Cancer and Cervical Cancer Incidence with Income and Education among Whites and Blacks," *Journal of the National Cancer Institute* 65 (1986): 515–28.

65. Ames, Magaw, and Gold, "Ranking Possible Carcinogenic Factors."

66. Quoted in R. Gillette, "Fallout Hazards Believed Less Than Many Suspected," *Los Angeles Times*, November 3, 1988.

67. A. I. Holleb, "Immunotherapy: A Realistic Appraisal" (interview with C. McKann), *CA* 30 (1980): 286–93.

68. Ross, "Avoidable Nondietary Risk Factors."

69. Ramming and Haskell, "Colorectal Malignancies."

70. Caporaso, "Lung Cancer and the Debrisoquine Metabolic Phenotype."

71. J. E. Bishop, "Drug Urged for Preventing Breast Cancer," *Wall Street Journal*, April 3, 1991.

72. J. Hooper, "The Asbestos Mess," *New York Times*, November 25, 1990.

73. American Cancer Society, *Cancer Rates and Risks*.

74. M. Stern, "The Recent Decline in Ischemic Heart Disease Mortality," *Annals of Internal Medicine* 91 (1979): 630–40.

75. S. Pell and W. Fayerweather, "Trends in the Incidence of Myocardial Infarction and Associated Mortality and Morbidity in a Large Employed Population, 1975–1983," *New England Journal of Medicine* 312 (1985): 1005–11.

76. J. K. Ockene et al., "The Relationship of Smoking Cessation to Coronary Heart Disease and Lung Cancer in the Multiple Risk Factor Intervention Trial (MRFIT)," *American Journal of Public Health* 80 (1990): 954–58.

Chapter 5

1. Quoted in D. Goldman, "The Mind over the Body," *New York Times Magazine*, September 27, 1987, p. 39.

2. C. Thomas, ed., *The Precursors Study: A Prospective Study of a Cohort of Medical Students*, vol. 5 (Baltimore: Johns Hopkins University Press, 1983).

3. O. C. Simonton, S. Matthews-Simonton, and J. L. Creighton, *Getting Well Again* (New York: Bantam, 1978).

4. L. Le Shan, *You Can Fight for Life: Emotional Factors in the Causation of Cancer* (New York: M. Evans, 1977).

5. S. Sontag, *Illness as Metaphor* (New York: Farrar, Straus, and Giroux, 1978).

6. Ibid., p. 21.

7. N. Cousins, *Anatomy of an Illness as Perceived by the Patient* (New York: Norton, 1979).

8. Ibid., p. 44.

9. Simonton, Matthews-Simonton, and Creighton, *Getting Well Again*, p. 10.

10. W. G. Glenn and R. E. Becker, "Individual v. Group Housing in Mice: Immunological Response to Time-Phased Injections," *Physiological Zoology* 42 (1969): 411–16.

11. Ibid., p. 414.

12. M. E. Lippman, "Psychosocial Factors and the Hormonal Regulation of Tumor Growth," in *Behavior and Cancer,* ed. S. Levy (San Francisco: Jossey-Bass, 1985), pp. 134–47.

13. M. Stein, R. C. Schiavi, and M. Camerino, "Influence of Brain and Behavior on the Immune System," *Science* 191 (1976): 435–40.

14. S. J. Schleifer, S. E. Keller, and M. Stein, "Central Nervous System Mechanisms and Immunity: Implications for Tumor Response," in *Behavior and Cancer,* pp. 120–33, at p. 122.

15. M. E. Lippman, "Clinical Implications of Glucocorticoid Receptors in Human Leukemia," *Cancer Research* 38 (1978): 4251–56.

16. L. R. Derogatis, M. D. Abeloff, and N. Melisartos, "Psychological Coping and Survival Time in Metastatic Breast Cancer," *Journal of the American Medical Association* 242 (1979): 1504–8.

17. G. N. Rogentine et al., "Psychological Factors in the Prognosis of Malignant Melanoma: A Prospective Study," *Psychosomatic Medicine* 41 (1979): 647–55.

18. S. Greer, T. Morris, and K. W. Pettigale, "Psychological Response to Breast Cancer: Effects on Outcome," *Lancet* 2 (1979): 785–87.

19. B. R. Cassileth et al., "Psychosocial Correlates of Survival in Advanced Malignant Disease?" *New England Journal of Medicine* 312 (1985): 1551–55.

20. P. P. Vitaliano, P. A. Lipscomb, and J. E. Carr, Letter to the Editor, *New England Journal of Medicine* 313 (1985): 1355.

21. H. P. Greenwald, "The Specificity of Quality-of-Life Measures among the Seriously Ill," *Medical Care* 25 (1987): 642–51.

22. M. Bergner et al., "The Sickness Impact Profile: Conceptual Formulation and Methodological Development of a Health Status Index," *International Journal of Health Service* 6 (1976): 393–415.

23. H. Selye, "Stress, Cancer, and the Mind," in *Cancer, Stress, and Death,* 2nd ed., ed. S. B. Day (New York: Plenum, 1984), pp. 11–19, at p. 12.

24. Ibid., pp. 15–16.

Chapter 6

1. J. T. Patterson, *The Dread Disease: Cancer and Modern American Culture* (Cambridge, Mass.: Harvard University Press, 1987), see especially pp. 72–73, 174–76.

2. American Cancer Society, *Cancer Facts and Figures, 1987* (New York: American Cancer Society, 1987), p. 3.

3. M. L. Berman et al., "Carcinoma of the Uterine Cervix," in *Cancer Treatment,* 2nd ed., ed. C. M. Haskell (Philadelphia: Saunders, 1985), pp. 429–42.

4. B. Stenkvist et al., "Papanicolaou Smear Screening and Cervical Cancer: What Can You Expect?" *Journal of the American Medical Association* 252 (1984): 1423–26.

5. N. E. Day, "The Effect of Cervical Cancer Screening in Scandinavia," *Obstetrics and Gynecology* 63 (1984): 714–18.

6. S. Shapiro, "Evidence on Screening for Breast Cancer from a Randomized Trial," *Cancer* 39 (1977): 2772–82.

7. D. M. Eddy, "Screening for Cancer of the Colon and Rectum," paper presented at the Second International Symposium on Colorectal Cancer, Washington, D.C., 1981; V. A. Gilbertson, "Proctosigmoidoscopy and Polypectomy in Reducing the Incidence of Rectal Cancer," *Cancer* 34 (1974): 936–39.

8. Eddy, "Screening for Cancer of the Colon"; R. E. Hertz, "Value of Periodic Examinations in Detecting Cancer of the Colon and Rectum," *Postgraduate Medicine* 27 (1960): 290–94.

9. W. K. Frankenburg and B. W. Camp, eds., *Periodic Screening Tests* (Springfield, Ill.: Thomas, 1975); P. Cole and A. S. Morrison, "Basic Issues in Population Screening for Cancer," *Journal of the National Cancer Institute* 64 (1980): 1263–72.

10. Patterson, *The Dread Disease,* p. 174.

11. R. A. Malt, "Treatment of Pancreatic Cancer," *Journal of the American Medical Association* 250 (1983): 1433–37, at 1433.

12. W. F. Taylor et al., "Some Results of Screening for Early Lung Cancer," *Cancer* 47 (1981): 1114–20.

13. J. B. Flehinger and M. Kimmel, "The Natural History of Lung Cancer in a Periodically Screened Population," *Biometrics* 43 (1987): 127–44.

14. G. P. Sarna et al., "Lung Cancer," in *Cancer Treatment,* pp. 180–211.

15. J. B. de Kernion, "Cancer of the Prostate," in *Cancer Treatment,* pp. 352–66.

16. A. M. Foltz and J. L. Kelsey, "The Annual Pap Test: A Dubious Policy Success," *Milbank Memorial Fund Quarterly* 56 (1978): 426–61.

17. W. Bogdanich, "Lax Laboratories: The Pap Test Misses Much Cervical Cancer through Lab's Errors," *Wall Street Journal,* November 2, 1987, sec. A, p. 1.

18. H. P. Greenwald, S. W. Becker, and M. C. Nevitt, "Delay and Non-compliance in Cancer Detection: A Behavioral Perspective for Health Planners," *Milbank Memorial Fund Quarterly* 56 (1978): 212–30.

19. G. T. Peck and J. S. Gallo, "Culpability for Delay in Treatment of Cancer," *American Journal of Cancer* 33 (1938): 443–62.

20. H. B. Makover, "Patient and Physician Delay in Cancer Diagnosis: Medical Aspects," *Journal of Chronic Diseases* 16 (1963): 419–26.

21. S. Shapiro, P. Strax, and L. Venet, "Periodic Breast Cancer Screening in Reducing Mortality from Breast Cancer," *Journal of the American Medical Association* 215 (1971): 1777–85.

22. H. P. Greenwald, "HMO Membership, Copayment, and Initiation of Care for Cancer: A Study of Working Adults," *American Journal of Public Health* 77 (1987): 461–66.

23. P. Greenwald et al., "Estimated Effect of Breast Self-Examination and Routine Physical Examination on Breast Cancer Mortality," *New England Journal of Medicine* 299 (1978): 271–73.

24. A. R. Feinstein, D. M. Sosin, and C. K. Wells, "The Will Rogers Phenomenon: Stage Migration and New Diagnostic Techniques as a Source of Misleading Statistics for Survival in Cancer," *New England Journal of Medicine* 312 (1985): 1604–8.

Chapter 7

1. M. Weber, "Class, Status, and Party," in *From Max Weber: Essays in Sociology,* ed. H. Gerth and C. W. Mills (New York: Oxford University Press, 1946).

2. R. W. Hodge and D. J. Treiman, "Class Identification in the United States," *American Journal of Sociology* 75 (1968): 535–47.

3. R. Sennett and J. Cobb, *The Hidden Injuries of Class* (New York: Knopf, 1972).

4. R. Dahrendorf, *Class and Class Conflict in Industrial Society* (Stanford, Calif.: Stanford University Press, 1959).

5. R. Venneman and L. W. Cannon, *The American Perception of Class* (Philadelphia: Temple University Press, 1987).

6. E. W. Bakke, *Citizens without Work: A Study of the Effects of Unemployment upon Workers' Social Relations and Practices* (New Haven, Conn.: Yale University Press, 1940), p. 80.

7. M. Janowitz, *The Professional Soldier* (New York: Free Press, 1960).

8. E. Kitagawa and P. Hauser, "Trends in Differential Fertility and Mortality in a Metropolis—Chicago," in *Contributions to Urban Sociology,* ed. E. Burgess and D. Bogue (Chicago: University of Chicago Press, 1964), pp. 59–85.

9. P. Townsend and N. Davidson, eds., *The Black Report* (London: Penguin, 1982).

10. Ibid.

11. D. T. Wigle and Y. Mao, *Mortality by Income Level in Urban Canada* (Ottawa: Health and Welfare, Canada, Health Protection Branch, 1980).

12. J. M. Axtel and M. H. Myers, "Contrasts in Survival of Black and White Cancer Patients, 1960–73," *Journal of the National Cancer Institute* 60 (1978): 1209–15.

13. J. L. Young, L. G. Ries, and E. S. Pollack, "Cancer Patient Survival among Ethnic Groups in the United States," *Journal of the National Cancer Institute* 73 (1984): 341–52.

14. A. Nomura et al., "Racial Survival Patterns for Lung Cancer in Hawaii," *Cancer* 48 (1981): 1265–71; L. Le Marchand, L. Kolenel, and A. Nomura, "Relationship of Ethnicity and Other Prognostic Factors to Breast Cancer Survival Patterns in Hawaii," *Journal of the National Cancer Institute* 73 (1984): 1259–65.

15. G. Linden, "The Influence of Social Class in the Survival of Cancer Patients," *American Journal of Public Health* 59 (1969): 267–74.

16. L. Lipworth, T. Abelin, and R. R. Connelly, "Socioeconomic Factors in the Prognosis of Cancer Patients," *Journal of Chronic Diseases* 23 (1970): 105–16.

17. J. Berg, R. Ross, and H. B. Latourette, "Economic Status and Survival of Cancer Patients," *Cancer* 39 (1977): 467–77.

18. T. N. Chirikos, N. A. Reihes, and M. L. Moeschberger, "Economic Differences in Cancer Survival: A Multivariate Analysis," *Journal of Chronic Diseases* 37 (1984): 183–93.

19. T. N. Chirikos, "Economic Status and Survivorship in Digestive System Cancers," *Cancer* 56 (1985): 210–17.

20. H. H. Dayal, L. Polissar, and S. Dahlberg, "Race, Socioeconomic Status, and Other Prognostic Factors for Survival from Prostate Cancer," *Journal of the National Cancer Institute* 74 (1985): 1001–6.

21. M. T. Bassett and N. Krieger, "Social Class and Black-White Differences in Breast Cancer Survival," *American Journal of Public Health* 76 (1986): 12.

22. H. P. Freeman, "Cancer in the Economically Disadvantaged," *Cancer* 64 (supp.) (1989): 324–34, at 331.

23. W. F. Page and A. J. Kuntz, "Race and Socioeconomic Factors in Cancer Survival: A Comparison of Veterans Administration Results with Selected Studies," *Cancer* 45 (1980): 1029–40.

Chapter 8

1. D. Mechanic, "The Organization of Medical Practice and Practice Orientations among Physicians in Prepaid and Nonprepaid Primary Care Settings," *Medical Care* 13 (1975): 189–204.

2. L. D. Brown, *Politics and Health Care Organization: HMOs as Federal Policy* (Washington, D.C.: Brookings Institution, 1983), p. 53.

3. C. C. Cutting, "Historical Development and Operating Concepts," in *The*

Kaiser Permanente Medical Care Program: A Symposium, ed. A. R. Somers (New York: Commonwealth Fund, 1971).

4. S. Fleming, "Anatomy of the Kaiser Permanente Program," in *The Kaiser Permanente Medical Care Program,* pp. 24, 25.

5. Brown, *Politics and Health Care Organization,* pp. 103–4.

6. Ibid., pp. 115–16.

7. P. Starr, *The Social Transformation of American Medicine* (New York: Basic Books, 1982), see book 2, chaps. 1 and 2.

8. Brown, *Politics and Health Care Organization,* p. 104.

9. E. Freidson, *Doctoring Together: A Study of Professional Social Control* (Chicago: Elsevier, 1975), pp. 61–62.

10. Ibid., p. 86.

11. H. S. Luft, "How Do Health-Maintenance Organizations Achieve Their 'Savings'?" *New England Journal of Medicine* 298 (1978): 1342.

12. Brown, *Politics and Health Care Organization,* p. 132.

13. Ibid., p. 133.

14. R. H. Brook et al., "Does Free Care Improve Adults' Health? Results from a Randomized Controlled Trial," *New England Journal of Medicine* 309 (1983): 1426–34.

15. W. G. Manning et al., "A Controlled Trial of the Effect of a Prepaid Group Practice on the Use of Services," *New England Journal of Medicine* 310 (1984): 1505–10.

16. J. E. Ware, W. H. Rogers, and A. R. Davies, "Comparison of Health Outcomes at a Health Maintenance Organization with Those of Fee-for-Service Care," *Lancet* 1 (1986): 1017–22.

17. J. McKusker, A. M. Stoddard, and A. A. Sorensen, "Do HMOs Reduce Hospitalization of Terminal Cancer Patients?" *Inquiry* 25 (1988): 263–70.

18. A. M. Francis, L. Polissar, and A. B. Lorenz, "Care of Patients with Colorectal Cancer: A Comparison of a Health Maintenance Organization and Fee-for-Service Practices," *Medical Care* 22 (1984): 418–29.

19. Group Health Cooperative of Puget Sound, *We Knew We Could Do It: An Oral History of the Origins and Early Years of Group Health Cooperative of Puget Sound* (Seattle: Group Health Cooperative of Puget Sound, 1983).

20. D. Paton, "Can Group Health, Seattle's Reigning Medical Center, Fight Off Its Imitators without Compromising Its Mission?" *Seattle Weekly,* November 14–20, 1984, pp. 39–45.

21. D. C. Cherkin, L. Grothaus, and E. H. Wagner, "The Effect of Office Visit Copayments on Preventive Care Services in an HMO," *Inquiry* 27 (1990): 24–38; and "The Effect of Office Visit Copayments on Utilization in a Health Maintenance Organization," *Medical Care* 27 (1989): 669–79.

Chapter 9

1. G. L. Gaumer, "Regulating Health Professionals: A Review of the Empirical Literature," *Milbank Memorial Fund Quarterly* 62 (1984): 380–416.

2. S. S. Mick and J. L. Worobey, "Foreign and United States Medical Graduates in Practice," *Medical Care* 22 (1984): 1014–25.

3. M. S. Baker, L. G. Kessler, and R. C. Smucker, "Site-Specific Treatment Costs for Cancer: An Analysis of the Medicare Continuous History Sample File," in *Cancer Care and Costs: DRGs and Beyond,* ed. R. M. Scheffler and N. C. Andrews (Ann Arbor, Mich.: Health Administration Press, 1989), pp. 127–38.

4. B. S. Stoll, "What Is Overtreatment in Cancer?" in *Costs versus Benefits in Cancer Care,* ed. B. S. Stoll (Baltimore: Johns Hopkins University Press, 1988).

5. L. D. Schaeffer and B. S. Gould, "Cancer Care and Cost: The Blue Cross of California Approach," in *Cancer Care and Costs,* pp. 181–93, at p. 185.

6. C. R. Whitney, "British Health Service, Much Beloved but Inadequate, Is Facing Changes," *New York Times,* June 9, 1991, sec. 1, p. 11.

7. D. Callahan, *What Kind of Life: The Limits of Medical Progress* (New York: Simon and Schuster, 1990).

Appendix A

1. D. M. McNair, M. Lorr, and L. F. Doppleman, *EITS Manual for the Profile of Mood States* (San Diego: Educational and Industrial Testing Service, 1981).

2. M. Bergner et al., "The Sickness Impact Profile: Validation of a Health Status Measure," *Medical Care* 14 (1976): 57.

3. R. Melzack, "The McGill Pain Questionnaire: Major Properties and Scoring Methods," *Pain* 1 (1975): 277–99.

4. E. M. Smith, A. M. Francis, and L. Polissar, "The Effect of Breast Self-Exam Practices and Physician Examinations on Extent of Disease at Diagnosis," *Preventive Medicine* 9 (1980): 409–17.

5. J. L. Young, Jr., C. L. Percy, and A. J. Asire, *Cancer Incidence and Mortality in the United States, 1973–1977,* NCI Monograph no. 57 (Bethesda, Md.: National Cancer Institute, 1981).

6. J. W. Horm, A. J. Asire, and J. L. Young, Jr., *SEER Program: Cancer Incidence and Mortality in the United States, 1973–1981,* USDHHS Pub. no. (NIH) 85-1837 (Washington, D.C.: U.S. Government Printing Office, 1984).

7. L. G. Riles, E. S. Pollack, and J. H. Young, Jr., "Cancer Patient Survival: Surveillance, Epidemiology, and End Results Program, 1973–79," *Journal of the National Cancer Institute* 70 (1983): 693–707.

Appendix B

1. L. A. Aday and S. M. Shortell, "Indicators and Predictors of Health Services Utilization," in *Introduction to Health Services,* 3rd ed., ed. S. J. Williams and P. R. Torrens (New York: Wiley, 1988), pp. 51–82.

2. D. R. Cox, "Regression Models and Life Tables" (with discussion), *Journal of the Royal Statistical Society* 34 (1972): 187–220.

3. S. P. Joyner, ed., *SUGI Supplemental Library User's Guide* (Cary, N.C.: SAS Institute, 1983).

4. J. D. Kalbfleish and R. L. Prentice, *The Statistical Analysis of Failure Time Data* (New York: Wiley, 1980).

5. "SEER Program Summary Staging Guide," unpublished program document, USDHHS, National Cancer Institute, 1977.

6. O. D. Duncan and P. M. Blau, *The American Occupational Structure* (New York: Wiley, 1967).

7. Puget Sound Health Systems Agency, *Managed Health Care Plans: A Directory of HMOs and PPOs Offering Health Plans in Washington State* (Seattle: Puget Sound Health Systems Agency, 1985).

Index

Designer: Barbara Jellow
Compositor: Keystone Typesetting, Inc.
Text: 10/13 Galliard
Display: Galliard
Printer: Maple-Vail Book Mfg. Group
Binder: Maple-Vail Book Mfg. Group

DATE DUE			
MAR 2 4 1998			
MAY 0 2 2000			